S0-EGP-917

Acupressure Guide

Alleviate Headaches, Neck and Joint Pain, Anxiety Attacks, and Other Ailments

by

Dr. Aaron Stein

Second Edition

MobileReference.com
eBooks and Reference Literature for Mobile Devices and electronic Readers™

Second edition, April, 2009
First published December, 2004

ISBN-13: 978-1-60778-778-5
Library of Congress Control Number: 2009926678

To see all Acupressure, Yoga, Diet, and other Health-related software for smartphones, iPhone and other mobile devices please visit
WWW.SOUNDTELLS.COM

SoundTells®. Software for Health™.

Printed in Canada

Contents

General Directions

- ❏ Use deep firm pressure to massage every point.
- ❏ Usually acupressure points are more sensitive than surrounding area.
- ❏ The massage duration indicated with point description is only an approximation. Massage every point until a numbing feeling is produced.
- ❏ You do not need to massage all active points included in the exercise. Some active points produce stronger effect than others. You may choose to limit the treatment to massaging these high potency points only.
- ❏ You can repeat active points massage as often as you want. There is no limit on number of treatments per day.
- ❏ When applying a deep pressure, the active point is expected to hurt initially. In this case reduce the pressure to a "comfortably" painful level and persist with massaging the active point. Increase the pressure as the initial painful sensation begins to subside. Continue the massage until a numbing feeling is produced
- ❏ When massaging acupressure points sit comfortably or lie down, close your eyes and breathe deeply.
- ❏ It is not necessary to massage points on your own, you can ask somebody else to massage your active points.
- ❏ An example of stimulation of active point Li4 is shown below. Point Li4 is located between thumb and index finger. Apply firm deep strokes of pressure in upward direction:

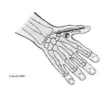 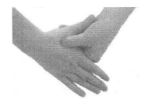

GENERAL DIRECTIONS

Warning

This acupressure guide is not a substitution for a qualified medical advice. If you do not know what is causing the pain or other symptom consult a medical doctor before you start treating yourself.

How Acupressure Works

Acupressure and acupuncture share the same active points (also called trigger points). The ancient Chinese developed system of active points stimulation over 5,000 years ago. The active points are located on imaginary lines called meridians. Accordingly, the points are referred to by the meridian they are located on and a consecutive number of the point on that meridian.

Commonly used meridian names and abbreviations

Meridian Names	Abbreviations Used In This Book	Other Abbreviations
Urinary Bladder	B	BL
Conception Vessel (also Ren Meridian)	CV	RN
Gall Bladder	GB	GB
Governor Vessel (also Du Meridian)	GV	DU
Heart	H	HT
Kidney	K	K
Large Intestine	Li	LI
Liver	Liv	LR
Lung	Lu	
Pericardium	P	PC
Small Intestine	Si	SI
Stomach	St	ST
Spleen	Sp	SP
Triplewarmer (also Sanjiao Meridian)	TW	SJ

The ancient Chinese believed that life energy chi (pronounced *chee*) flows through these meridians. In a healthy person, the energy flow trough meridians is unobstructed. The blockade of chi flow results in an illness. The Chinese believed that active points stimulation clears the meridians and improves the flow of energy.

The western medical science only begins to understand the mechanisms responsible for positive effects of active points stimulation. Stimulation of active points is thought to lead to increased release of endorphins. Endorphin is a natural body painkiller. Endorphin and morphine are

HOW ACCUPRESSURE WORKS

chemically different molecules but, by coincidence, they have very similar 3-dimensional shape. This similarity in shape allows morphine to bind the endorphin receptor, reduce pain, and induce feeling of happiness. Thus endorphin released by acupressure stimulation may lead to relaxation and normalization of body functions.

Headache And Migraine:
Frontal Headache

Headache is often due to build-up of stress and tension. Acupressure is an effective way to relieve painful sensation associated these conditions. Treat as soon as first sign of headache appear. Do not wait for full blown headache.

Sit comfortably or lie down, close your eyes and breathe deeply when massaging the active points.

STEP 1: Acupressure Point B2 - *Start with a less painful side*

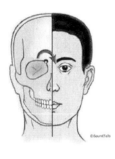

Location: with the tip of your thumb or index finger probe the area where the bridge of the nose meets the ridge of the eyebrows until you feel a slight dip.

Direction: apply firm deep strokes of pressure in downward direction. The initial painful sensation will soon begin to subside.

Duration: 1 min

STEP 2: Acupressure point B2 - *Switch to a more painful side*

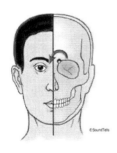

Location: with the tip of your thumb or index finger probe the area where the bridge of the nose meets the ridge of the eyebrows until you feel a slight dip.

Direction: apply firm deep strokes of pressure in downward direction. The initial painful sensation will soon begin to subside.

Duration: 1 min

STEP 3: Acupressure Point Yin Tang

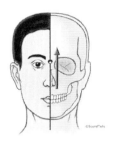

Location: with the tip of your thumb or index finger probe the area midway between the medial end of the two eyebrows as indicated on the picture until you feel a slight dip.

Direction: apply firm deep strokes of pressure in upward direction. The initial painful sensation will soon begin to subside

Duration: 1 min

STEP 4: Acupressure Point GB14 - *Start with a less painful side*

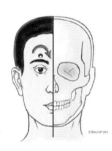

Location: with the tip of your index finger probe the area directly up from the pupil of the eye when looking straight ahead, approximately one finger-width above the eyebrow, until you feel a slight dip.

Direction: apply firm deep strokes of pressure in downward direction. The initial painful sensation will soon begin to subside.

Duration: 1 min

STEP 5: Acupressure Point GB14 - *Switch to a more painful side*

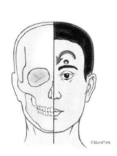

Location: with the tip of your index finger probe the area directly up from the pupil of the eye when looking straight ahead, approximately one finger-width above the eyebrow, until you feel a slight dip.

Direction: apply firm deep strokes of pressure in downward direction. The initial painful sensation will soon begin to subside.

Duration: 1 min

STEP 6: Acupressure Point Li4 - This point is forbidden for pregnant women - *Start with a less painful side*

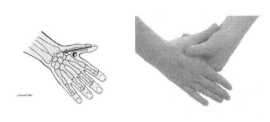

Location: between thumb and index finger as indicated on the picture.

Direction: apply firm deep strokes of pressure in upward direction. The initial painful sensation will soon begin to subside.

Duration: 2 min

STEP 7: Acupressure Point Li4 - This point is forbidden for pregnant women - *Switch to a more painful side*

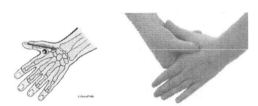

Location: between thumb and index finger as indicated on the picture.

Direction: apply firm deep strokes of pressure in upward direction. The initial painful sensation will soon begin to subside.

Duration: 2 min

STEP 8: Acupressure Point St36 - This point is forbidden for pregnant women - *Start with a less painful side*

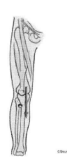

Location: with the tip of your index finger probe the area on the front side of a leg below the knee until you feel a slight dip.

Direction: apply firm deep strokes of pressure in downward direction. The initial painful sensation will soon begin to subside.

Duration: 1 min

STEP 9: Acupressure Point St36 - This point is forbidden for pregnant women - *Switch to a more painful side*

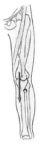

Location: with the tip of your index finger probe the area on the front side of a leg below the knee until you feel a slight dip.

Direction: apply firm deep strokes of pressure in downward direction. The initial painful sensation will soon begin to subside.

Duration: 1 min

STEP 10: Acupressure Point Liv3 - *Start with a less painful side*

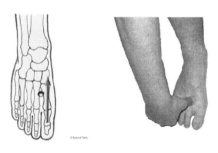

Location: on the top of the foot in the webbing between the big toe and the second toe.

Direction: apply firm deep strokes of pressure in upward direction. The initial painful sensation will soon begin to subside.

Duration: 1 min

STEP 11: Acupressure Point Liv3 - *Switch to a more painful side*

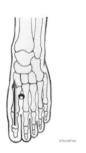 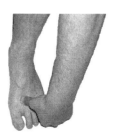

Location: on the top of the foot in the webbing between the big toe and the second toe.

Direction: apply firm deep strokes of pressure in upward direction. The initial painful sensation will soon begin to subside.

Duration: 1 min

Headache In The Back Of The Head

Headache is often due to build-up of stress and tension. Acupressure is an effective way to relieve painful sensation associated these conditions. Treat as soon as first sign of headache appear. Do not wait for full blown headache.

Sit comfortably or lie down, close your eyes and breathe deeply when massaging the active points.

STEP 1: Acupressure Point Li4 - This point is forbidden for pregnant women - *Start with a less painful side*

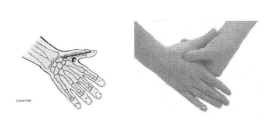

Location: between thumb and index finger as indicated on the picture.

Direction: apply firm deep strokes of pressure in upward direction. The initial painful sensation will soon begin to subside.

Duration: 2 min

STEP 2: Acupressure Point Li4 - This point is forbidden for pregnant women - *Switch to a more painful side*

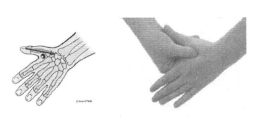

Location: between thumb and index finger as indicated on the picture.

Direction: apply firm deep strokes of pressure in upward direction. The initial painful sensation will soon begin to subside.

Duration: 2 min

14

STEP 3: Acupressure Point St3 - *Start with a less painful side*

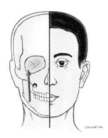

Location: below the cheekbone, directly down from the pupil of the eye.

Direction: apply firm deep strokes of pressure in upward direction against the bottom edge of the cheekbone. The initial painful sensation will soon begin to subside.

Duration: 1 min

STEP 4: Acupressure Point St3 - *Switch to a more painful side*

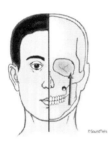

Location: below the cheekbone, directly down from the pupil of the eye.

Direction: apply firm deep strokes of pressure in upward direction against the bottom edge of the cheekbone. The initial painful sensation will soon begin to subside.

Duration: 1 min

STEP 5: Acupressure Point GB20 - *Start with a less painful side*

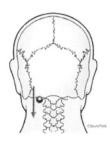

Location: just below the base of the scull, in the depression between the two major neck muscles.

Direction: apply firm deep strokes of pressure in downward direction.

Duration: 1 min

STEP 6: Acupressure Point GB20 - *Switch to a more painful side*

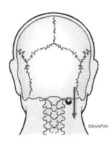

Location: just below the base of the scull, in the depression between the two major neck muscles.

Direction: apply firm deep strokes of pressure in downward direction.

Duration: 1 min

STEP 7: Acupressure Point GV16

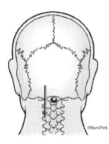

Location: in the back of the head, in the large depression under the base of the skull.

Direction: apply firm deep strokes of pressure in downward direction. The initial painful sensation will soon begin to subside.

Duration: 2 min

STEP 8: Acupressure Point St36 - **This point is forbidden for pregnant women** - *Start with a less painful side*

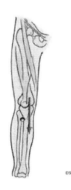

Location: with the tip of your index finger probe the area on the front side of a leg below the knee until you feel a slight dip.

Direction: apply firm deep strokes of pressure in downward direction. The initial painful sensation will soon begin to subside.

Duration: 1 min

STEP 9: Acupressure Point St36 - This point is forbidden for pregnant women - *Switch to a more painful side*

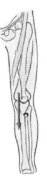

Location: with the tip of your index finger probe the area on the front side of a leg below the knee until you feel a slight dip.

Direction: apply firm deep strokes of pressure in downward direction. The initial painful sensation will soon begin to subside.

Duration: 1 min

Headache On The Side Of The Head

Headache is often due to build-up of stress and tension. Acupressure is an effective way to relieve painful sensation associated these conditions. Treat as soon as first sign of headache appear. Do not wait for full blown headache.

Sit comfortably or lie down, close your eyes and breathe deeply when massaging the active points.

STEP 1: Acupressure Point GB20 - *Start with a less painful side*

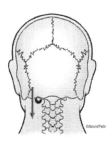

Location: just below the base of the scull, in the depression between the two major neck muscles.

Direction: apply firm deep strokes of pressure in downward direction.

Duration: 1 min

STEP 2: Acupressure Point GB20 - *Switch to a more painful side*

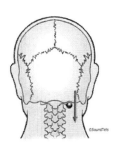

Location: just below the base of the scull, in the depression between the two major neck muscles.

Direction: apply firm deep strokes of pressure in downward direction.

Duration: 1 min

STEP 3: Acupressure Point Tai Yang - *Start with a less painful side*

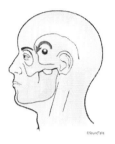

Location: in the large depression on the side of the head about 1 inch away from the end of the eyebrow.

Direction: massage in circular motions back to front. The initial painful sensation will soon begin to subside

Duration: 1 min

STEP 4: Acupressure Point Tai Yang - *Switch to a more painful side*

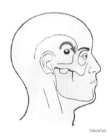

Location: in the large depression on the side of the head about 1 inch away from the end of the eyebrow.

Direction: massage in circular motions back to front. The initial painful sensation will soon begin to subside

Duration: 1 min

STEP 5: Acupressure Point St3 - *Start with a less painful side*

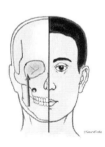

Location: below the cheekbone, directly down from the pupil of the eye.

Direction: apply firm deep strokes of pressure in upward direction against the bottom edge of the cheekbone. The initial painful sensation will soon begin to subside.

Duration: 1 min

STEP 6: Acupressure Point St3 - *Switch to a more painful side*

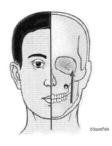

Location: below the cheekbone, directly down from the pupil of the eye.

Direction: apply firm deep strokes of pressure in upward direction against the bottom edge of the cheekbone. The initial painful sensation will soon begin to subside.

Duration: 1 min

STEP 7: Acupressure Point TW5 - *Start with a less painful side*

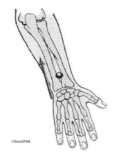

Location: on the back of the arm, in the depression between the two bones, three finger-width above the wrist crease.

Direction: apply firm deep strokes of pressure in upward direction. The initial painful sensation will soon begin to subside

Duration: 2 min

STEP 8: Acupressure Point TW5 - *Switch to a more painful side*

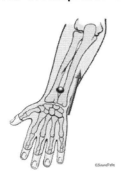

Location: on the back of the arm, in the depression between the two bones, three finger-width above the wrist crease.

Direction: apply firm deep strokes of pressure in upward direction. The initial painful sensation will soon begin to subside

Duration: 2 min

STEP 9: Acupressure Point St36 - This point is forbidden for pregnant women - *Start with a less painful side*

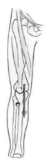

Location: with the tip of your index finger probe the area on the front side of a leg below the knee until you feel a slight dip.

Direction: apply firm deep strokes of pressure in downward direction. The initial painful sensation will soon begin to subside.

Duration: 1 min

STEP 10: Acupressure Point St36 - This point is forbidden for pregnant women - *Switch to a more painful side*

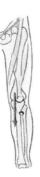

Location: with the tip of your index finger probe the area on the front side of a leg below the knee until you feel a slight dip.

Direction: apply firm deep strokes of pressure in downward direction. The initial painful sensation will soon begin to subside.

Duration: 1 min

STEP 11: Acupressure Point GB34 - *Start with a less painful side*

OUTSIDE

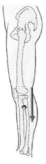

Location: bend you leg. With the tip of your index finger probe the area in front of and below the head of the outer leg bone until you feel a slight dip.

Direction: apply firm deep strokes of pressure in downward direction. The initial painful sensation will soon begin to subside.

Duration: 1 min

STEP 12: Acupressure Point GB34 - *Switch to a more painful side*

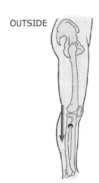

OUTSIDE

Location: bend you leg. With the tip of your index finger probe the area in front of and below the head of the outer leg bone until you feel a slight dip.

Direction: apply firm deep strokes of pressure in downward direction. The initial painful sensation will soon begin to subside.

Duration: 1 min

Headache On The Top Of The Head

Headache is often due to build-up of stress and tension. Acupressure is an effective way to relieve painful sensation associated these conditions. Treat as soon as first sign of headache appear. Do not wait for full blown headache.

Sit comfortably or lie down, close your eyes and breathe deeply when massaging the active points.

STEP 1: Acupressure Point GV20

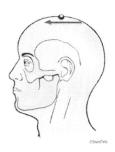

Location: with the tip of your index finger probe the area on the top of the head, where the line connecting the high points of your ears crosses the body midline until you feel a slight dip.

Direction: apply firm deep circular strokes of pressure in the forward direction. The initial painful sensation will soon begin to subside.

Duration: 2 min

STEP 2: Acupressure Point St3 - *Start with a less painful side*

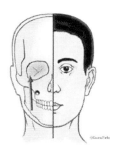

Location: below the cheekbone, directly down from the pupil of the eye.

Direction: apply firm deep strokes of pressure in upward direction against the bottom edge of the cheekbone. The initial painful sensation will soon begin to subside.

Duration: 1 min

STEP 3: Acupressure Point St3 - *Switch to a more painful side*

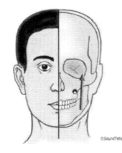

Location: below the cheekbone, directly down from the pupil of the eye.

Direction: apply firm deep strokes of pressure in upward direction against the bottom edge of the cheekbone. The initial painful sensation will soon begin to subside.

Duration: 1 min

STEP 4: Acupressure Point St36 - This point is forbidden for pregnant women - *Start with a less painful side*

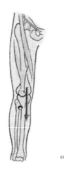

Location: with the tip of your index finger probe the area on the front side of a leg below the knee until you feel a slight dip.

Direction: apply firm deep strokes of pressure in downward direction. The initial painful sensation will soon begin to subside.

Duration: 1 min

STEP 5: Acupressure Point St36 - This point is forbidden for pregnant women - *Switch to a more painful side*

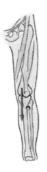

Location: with the tip of your index finger probe the area on the front side of a leg below the knee until you feel a slight dip.

Direction: apply firm deep strokes of pressure in downward direction. The initial painful sensation will soon begin to subside.

Duration: 1 min

24

STEP 6: Acupressure Point Liv3 - *Start with a less painful side*

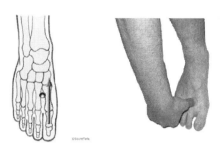

Location: on the top of the foot in the webbing between the big toe and the second toe.

Direction: apply firm deep strokes of pressure in upward direction. The initial painful sensation will soon begin to subside.

Duration: 1 min

STEP 7: Acupressure Point Liv3 - *Switch to a more painful side*

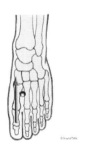 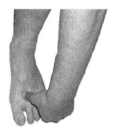

Location: on the top of the foot in the webbing between the big toe and the second toe.

Direction: apply firm deep strokes of pressure in upward direction. The initial painful sensation will soon begin to subside.

Duration: 1 min

Headache Behind The Eye

Headache is often due to build-up of stress and tension. Acupressure is an effective way to relieve painful sensation associated these conditions. Treat as soon as first sign of headache appear. Do not wait for full blown headache.

Sit comfortably or lie down, close your eyes and breathe deeply when massaging the active points.

STEP 1: Acupressure Point B1 - *Start with a less painful side*

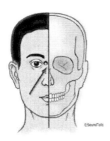

Location: just inside the inner corner of the eye.

Direction: press toward the bridge of the nose in upward strokes. The initial painful sensation will soon begin to subside

Duration: 1 min

STEP 2: Acupressure Point B1 - *Switch to a more painful side*

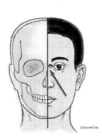

Location: just inside the inner corner of the eye.

Direction: press toward the bridge of the nose in upward strokes. The initial painful sensation will soon begin to subside

Duration: 1 min

HEADACHE AND MIGRAINE: *Pain In The Eye*

STEP 3: Acupressure Point Tai Yang - *Start with a less painful side*

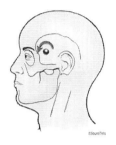

Location: in the large depression on the side of the head about 1 inch away from the end of the eyebrow.

Direction: massage in circular motions back to front. The initial painful sensation will soon begin to subside

Duration: 1 min

STEP4: Acupressure Point Tai Yang - *Switch to a more painful side*

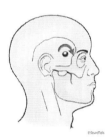

Location: in the large depression on the side of the head about 1 inch away from the end of the eyebrow.

Direction: massage in circular motions back to front. The initial painful sensation will soon begin to subside

Duration: 1 min

STEP 5: Acupressure Point Li4 - This point is forbidden for pregnant women - *Start with a less painful side*

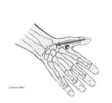 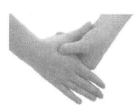

Location: between thumb and index finger as indicated on the picture.

Direction: apply firm deep strokes of pressure in upward direction. The initial painful sensation will soon begin to subside.

Duration: 2 min

STEP 6: Acupressure Point Li4 - This point is forbidden for pregnant women - *Switch to a more painful side*

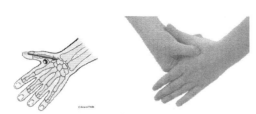

Location: between thumb and index finger as indicated on the picture.

Direction: apply firm deep strokes of pressure in upward direction. The initial painful sensation will soon begin to subside.

Duration: 2 min

STEP 7: Acupressure Point Liv3 - *Start with a less painful side*

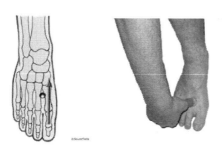

Location: on the top of the foot in the webbing between the big toe and the second toe.

Direction: apply firm deep strokes of pressure in upward direction. The initial painful sensation will soon begin to subside.

Duration: 1 min

STEP 8: Acupressure Point Liv3 - *Switch to a more painful side*

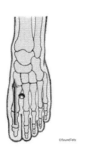 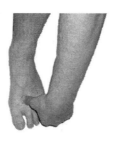

Location: on the top of the foot in the webbing between the big toe and the second toe.

Direction: apply firm deep strokes of pressure in upward direction. The initial painful sensation will soon begin to subside.

Duration: 1 min

Local Pain:
Pain In The Jaw

Acupressure is often successful in relieving jaw pain. Sit comfortably or lie down, close your eyes and breathe deeply when massaging the active points.

STEP 1: Acupressure Point Li4 - This point is forbidden for pregnant women - *Start with a less painful side*

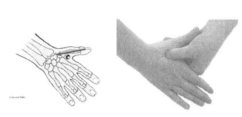

Location: between thumb and index finger as indicated on the picture.

Direction: apply firm deep strokes of pressure in upward direction. The initial painful sensation will soon begin to subside.

Duration: 2 min

STEP 2: Acupressure Point Li4 - This point is forbidden for pregnant women - *Switch to a more painful side*

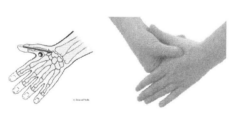

Location: between thumb and index finger as indicated on the picture.

Direction: apply firm deep strokes of pressure in upward direction. The initial painful sensation will soon begin to subside.

Duration: 2 min

STEP 3: Ear Point Si19, GB2, TW21 - *Start with a less painful side*

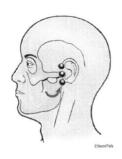

Location: Si9 is in the front of the ear hole in the hollow that becomes deeper when the mouth is open. GB2 is in the depression half finger-width below Si9. TW21 is in the depression half finger-width above Si9.

Direction: apply firm deep strokes of pressure. The initial painful sensation will soon begin to subside.

Duration: massage every point for about 1 min.

STEP 4: Ear Point Si19, GB2, TW21 - *Switch to a more painful side*

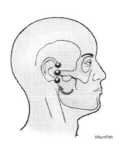

Location: Si9 is in the front of the ear hole in the hollow that becomes deeper when the mouth is open. GB2 is in the depression half finger-width below Si9. TW21 is in the depression half finger-width above Si9.

Direction: apply firm deep strokes of pressure. The initial painful sensation will soon begin to subside.

Duration: massage every point for about 1 min.

STEP 5: Acupressure Point St6 - *Start with a less painful side*

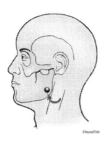

Location: on the muscle that bulges the teeth are clenched.

Direction: apply firm deep strokes of pressure into the jaw. The initial painful sensation will soon begin to subside.

Duration: 1 min

STEP 6: Acupressure Point St6 - *Switch to a more painful side*

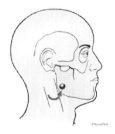

Location: on the muscle that bulges the teeth are clenched.

Direction: apply firm deep strokes of pressure into the jaw. The initial painful sensation will soon begin to subside.

Duration: 1 min

31

Toothache

STEP 1: Acupressure Point Li4 - This point is forbidden for pregnant women - *Start with a less painful side*

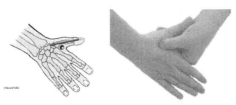

Location: between thumb and index finger as indicated on the picture.

Direction: apply firm deep strokes of pressure in upward direction. The initial painful sensation will soon begin to subside.

Duration: 2 min

STEP 2: Acupressure Point Li4 - This point is forbidden for pregnant women - *Switch to a more painful side*

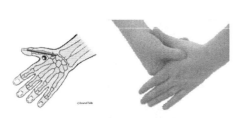

Location: between thumb and index finger as indicated on the picture.

Direction: apply firm deep strokes of pressure in upward direction. The initial painful sensation will soon begin to subside.

Duration: 2 min

STEP 3: Acupressure Point St6 - *Start with a less painful side*

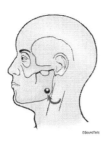

Location: on the muscle that bulges the teeth are clenched.

Direction: apply firm deep strokes of pressure into the jaw. The initial painful sensation will soon begin to subside.

Duration: 1 min

LOCAL PAIN: *Toothache*

STEP 4: Acupressure Point St6 - *Switch to a more painful side*

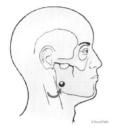

Location: on the muscle that bulges the teeth are clenched.

Direction: apply firm deep strokes of pressure into the jaw. The initial painful sensation will soon begin to subside.

Duration: 1 min

STEP 5: Acupressure Point St3 - *Start with a less painful side*

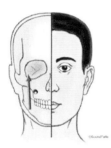

Location: below the cheekbone, directly down from the pupil of the eye.

Direction: apply firm deep strokes of pressure in upward direction against the bottom edge of the cheekbone. The initial painful sensation will soon begin to subside.

Duration: 1 min

STEP 6: Acupressure Point St3 - *Switch to a more painful side*

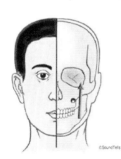

Location: below the cheekbone, directly down from the pupil of the eye.

Direction: apply firm deep strokes of pressure in upward direction against the bottom edge of the cheekbone. The initial painful sensation will soon begin to subside.

Duration: 1 min

Ear Pain

Sit comfortably or lie down, close your eyes and breathe deeply when massaging the active points.

STEP 1: Ear Point Si19, GB2, TW21 - *Start with a less painful side*

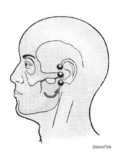

Location: Si9 is in the front of the ear hole in the hollow that becomes deeper when the mouth is open. GB2 is in the depression half finger-width below Si9. TW21 is in the depression half finger-width above Si9.

Direction: apply firm deep strokes of pressure. The initial painful sensation will soon begin to subside.

Duration: massage every point for about 1 min.

STEP 2: Ear Point Si19, GB2, TW21 - *Switch to a more painful side*

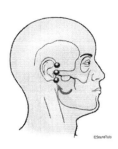

Location: Si9 is in the front of the ear hole in the hollow that becomes deeper when the mouth is open. GB2 is in the depression half finger-width below Si9. TW21 is in the depression half finger-width above Si9.

Direction: apply firm deep strokes of pressure. The initial painful sensation will soon begin to subside.

Duration: massage every point for about 1 min.

STEP 3: Acupressure Point TW17 - *Start with a less painful side*

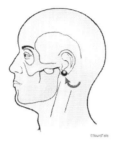

Location: in the hollow behind the ear lobe.

Direction: take a deep breath and slowly breathe out while holding this point.

Duration: 2 min

STEP 4: Acupressure Point TW17 - *Switch to a more painful side*

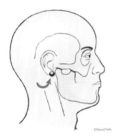

Location: in the hollow behind the ear lobe.

Direction: take a deep breath and slowly breathe out while holding this point.

Duration: 2 min

STEP 5: Acupressure Point GB20 - *Start with a less painful side*

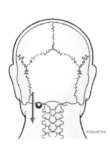

Location: just below the base of the scull, in the depression between the two major neck muscles.

Direction: apply firm deep strokes of pressure in downward direction.

Duration: 1 min

STEP 6: Acupressure Point GB20 - *Switch to a more painful side*

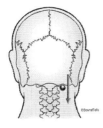

Location: just below the base of the scull, in the depression between the two major neck muscles.

Direction: apply firm deep strokes of pressure in downward direction.

Duration: 1 min

STEP 7: Acupressure Points K3 - This point is forbidden for pregnant women - *Start with a less painful side*

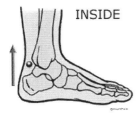

INSIDE

Location: in the hollow midway between inside anklebone and the Achilles tendon.

Direction: apply firm deep strokes of pressure in upward direction. The initial painful sensation will soon begin to subside.

Duration: 1 min

STEP 8: Acupressure Point K3 - This point is forbidden for pregnant women - *Switch to a more painful side*

INSIDE

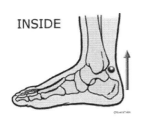

Location: in the hollow midway between inside anklebone and the Achilles tendon.

Direction: apply firm deep strokes of pressure in upward direction. The initial painful sensation will soon begin to subside.

Duration: 1 min

Neck Pain And Tension

Neck pain is commonly due to muscle tension. Acupressure is often successful in relieving neck pain. Sit comfortably or lie down, close your eyes and breathe deeply when massaging the active points.

STEP 1: Acupressure Point GB20 - *Start with a less painful side*

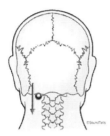

Location: just below the base of the scull, in the depression between the two major neck muscles.

Direction: apply firm deep strokes of pressure in downward direction.

Duration: 1 min

STEP 2: Acupressure Point GB20 - *Switch to a more painful side*

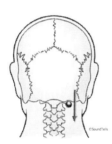

Location: just below the base of the scull, in the depression between the two major neck muscles.

Direction: apply firm deep strokes of pressure in downward direction.

Duration: 1 min

STEP 3: Acupressure Point B10 - *Start with a less painful side*

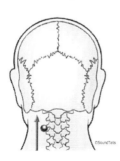

Location: halfway between the base of the skull and the base of the neck, on the edge of the trapezoid muscles.

Direction: apply firm deep strokes of pressure in upward direction. The initial painful sensation will soon begin to subside.

Duration: 1 min

STEP 4: Acupressure Point B10 - *Switch to a more painful side*

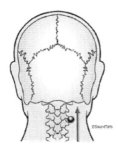

Location: halfway between the base of the skull and the base of the neck, on the edge of the trapezoid muscles.

Direction: apply firm deep strokes of pressure in upward direction. The initial painful sensation will soon begin to subside.

Duration: 1 min

STEP 5: Acupressure Point GB21 - *Start with a less painful side*

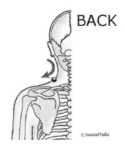

BACK

Location: on the top of the trapezoid muscle, directly up from the nipple.

Direction: apply firm deep strokes of pressure in downward direction. The initial painful sensation will soon begin to subside

Duration: 1 min

STEP 6: Acupressure Point GB21 - *Switch to a more painful side*

BACK

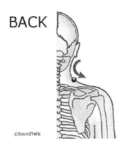

Location: on the top of the trapezoid muscle, directly up from the nipple.

Direction: apply firm deep strokes of pressure in downward direction. The initial painful sensation will soon begin to subside

Duration: 1 min

STEP 7: Acupressure Point Li4 - This point is forbidden for pregnant women - *Start with a less painful side*

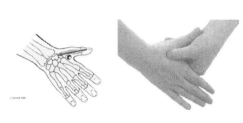

Location: between thumb and index finger as indicated on the picture.

Direction: apply firm deep strokes of pressure in upward direction. The initial painful sensation will soon begin to subside.

Duration: 2 min

STEP 8: Acupressure Point Li4 - This point is forbidden for pregnant women - *Switch to a more painful side*

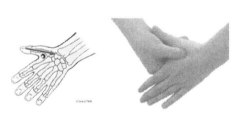

Location: between thumb and index finger as indicated on the picture.

Direction: apply firm deep strokes of pressure in upward direction. The initial painful sensation will soon begin to subside.

Duration: 2 min

STEP 9: Acupressure Point GV16

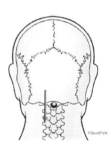

Location: in the back of the head, in the large depression under the base of the skull.

Direction: apply firm deep strokes of pressure in downward direction. The initial painful sensation will soon begin to subside.

Duration: 2 min

Shoulder Pain And Tension

Shoulder pain is a common problem. Acupressure is often successful in relieving shoulder pain. Sit comfortably or lie down, close your eyes and breathe deeply when massaging the local active points.

STEP 1: Acupressure Point GB21

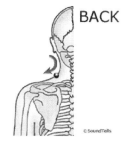

Location: on the top of the trapezoid muscle, directly up from the nipple.

Direction: apply firm deep strokes of pressure in downward direction. The initial painful sensation will soon begin to subside

Duration: 1 min

STEP 2: Acupressure Point TW15

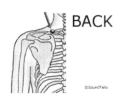

Location: on the top of the shoulder blade. To find the point go directly up from the nipple, around the top of the trapezoid muscle, and down to the top of the shoulder blade.

Direction: apply firm deep strokes of pressure in upward direction. The initial painful sensation will soon begin to subside

Duration: 1 min

STEP 3: Acupressure Point TW14

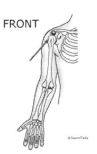

Location: in the front, in the hollow below the scapular bone and directly above the arm joint.

Direction: apply firm deep strokes of pressure in the direction of the scapular. The initial painful sensation will soon begin to subside.

Duration: 1 min

LOCAL PAIN: *Shoulder Pain And Tension*

STEP 4: Acupressure Point Li15

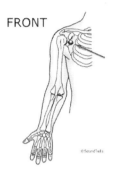

Location: in the front part of arm joint, in the anterior hollow formed when the arm is raised above the head. Lower the arm when massaging the point.

Direction: apply firm deep strokes of pressure in the direction of the joint. The initial painful sensation will soon begin to subside.

Duration: 1 min

STEP 5: Acupressure Point Li14

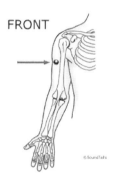

Location: on the outside of the arm, in the hollow where deltoid muscle is inserted into the humerus bone (the bone of the upper arm), about one third distance from the top of the shoulder to the elbow.

Direction: press directly into the humerus bone. The initial painful sensation will soon begin to subside

Duration: 1 min

STEP 6: Acupressure Point Li11

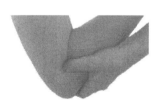

Location: bend your arm, press your thumb into the hollow located on the outer side of the arm, directly above the elbow, between the elbow joint (below) and the muscle (above).

Direction: apply firm deep strokes of pressure in the direction of the elbow joint. The initial painful sensation will soon begin to subside.

Duration: 1 min

LOCAL PAIN: *Shoulder Pain And Tension*

STEP 7: Acupressure Point B57

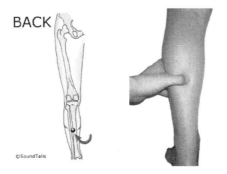

BACK

©SoundTells

Location: in the back of the leg, midway between the knee and the heel, at the bottom edge and between the two heads of the gastrocnemius muscle.

Direction: apply firm deep strokes of pressure in the direction of the bone. The initial painful sensation will soon begin to subside.

Duration: 1 min

Wrist Treatment

Wrist pain is often due to repetitive stress imposed on the wrist by computer related activity such as typing. Sometimes wrist pain is due to carpal tunnel syndrome. In this condition the inflamed tissue compresses the nerve inside the wrist (medial nerve). The nerve, in turn, releases chemical substances that inflame the tissue further. When treating this condition your goal is to stop the inflammation/compression cycle. Active points massage is an effective way to treat wrist pain. Often single 30 minutes treatment is sufficient to eliminate the pain for good. Treat active points for as long as you can or until numbing feeling is produced, as often as you can during the day.

Straitening the wrist at night facilitates healing by reducing pressure on the nerve. Some patients find it helpful to stabilize the wrist in straitened position by wearing the wrist splint.

Sit comfortably or lie down, close your eyes and breathe deeply when massaging the active points.

STEP 1: Acupressure Point P6

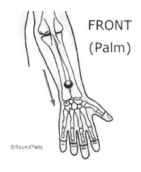

FRONT
(Palm)

Location: on the interior side of the arm, in the hollow between the bones of the forearm, three finger-width above the wrist crease.

Direction: apply firm deep strokes of pressure in the direction of the palm. The initial painful sensation will soon begin to subside

Duration: 3 min or more

43

STEP 2: Acupressure Point P7

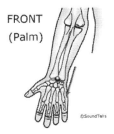

FRONT
(Palm)

Location: in the wrist, in the hollow between the bones of the forearm.

Direction: apply firm deep strokes of pressure in downward direction. The initial painful sensation will soon begin to subside.

Duration: 3 min or more

STEP 3: Acupressure Point TW5

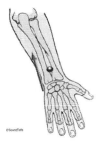

Location: on the back of the arm, in the depression between the two bones, three finger-width above the wrist crease.

Direction: apply firm deep strokes of pressure in upward direction. The initial painful sensation will soon begin to subside

Duration: 2 min

STEP 4: Acupressure Point TW4

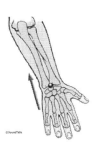

Location: on the back of the arm, in the center of the wrist crease.

Direction: apply firm deep strokes of pressure in upward direction. The initial painful sensation will soon begin to subside.

Duration: 2 min

STEP 5: Acupressure Point Li5

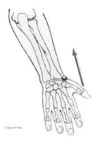

Location: in the wrist crease, near the thumb tendon. Move the thumb to feel the tendon movement.

Direction: apply firm deep strokes of pressure in upward direction. The initial painful sensation will soon begin to subside.

Duration: 2 min

STEP 6: Acupressure Point Si5

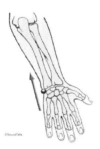

Location: in the wrist crease, in the hollow on the side of the wrist.

Direction: apply firm deep strokes of pressure in upward direction. The initial painful sensation will soon begin to subside.

Duration: 2 min

Hand Treatment

Acupressure is often successful in relieving hand pain. Sit comfortably or lie down, close your eyes and breathe deeply when massaging the active points.

STEP 1: Acupressure Point Li4 - This point is forbidden for pregnant women - *Start with a less painful side*

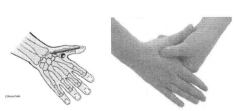

Location: between thumb and index finger as indicated on the picture.

Direction: apply firm deep strokes of pressure in upward direction. The initial painful sensation will soon begin to subside.

Duration: 2 min

STEP 2: Acupressure Point P6

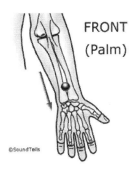

FRONT
(Palm)

Location: on the interior side of the arm, in the hollow between the bones of the forearm, three finger-width above the wrist crease.

Direction: apply firm deep strokes of pressure in the direction of the palm. The initial painful sensation will soon begin to subside

Duration: 3 min or more

46

STEP 3: Acupressure Point P7

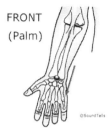

FRONT
(Palm)

Location: in the wrist, in the hollow between the bones of the forearm.

Direction: apply firm deep strokes of pressure in downward direction. The initial painful sensation will soon begin to subside.

Duration: 3 min

STEP 4: Acupressure Point TW4

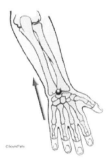

Location: on the back of the arm, in the center of the wrist crease.

Direction: apply firm deep strokes of pressure in upward direction. The initial painful sensation will soon begin to subside.

Duration: 2 min

STEP 5: Acupressure Point TW5

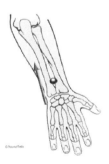

Location: on the back of the arm, in the depression between the two bones, three finger-width above the wrist crease.

Direction: apply firm deep strokes of pressure in upward direction. The initial painful sensation will soon begin to subside

Duration: 2 min

Lower Back Pain

Acupressure is often successful in relieving lower back pain. Sit comfortably or lie down, close your eyes and breathe deeply when massaging the active points.

STEP 1: Acupressure Points B23-B25 - *Start with a less painful side*

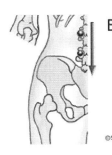

BAC

Location: B23 (top) - in the lower back, on the waist level, two finger-width away from the spine, in the hollow between vertebra.
B25 (bottom) - in the lower back, four finger-width below the waist level, two finger-width away from the spine, in the hollow between vertebra.

Direction: apply firm deep strokes of pressure in downward direction. If you are massaging these points yourself and cannot reach these points, lie back on a hard surface and position the tennis ball under the active points.

Duration: 1 min each point

STEP 2: Acupressure Point B23-25 - *Switch to a more painful side*

BACK

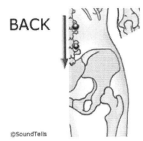

Location: B23 (top) - in the lower back, on the waist level, two finger-width away from the spine, in the hollow between vertebra.
B25 (bottom) - in the lower back, four finger-width below the waist level, two finger-width away from the spine, in the hollow between vertebra.

Direction: apply firm deep strokes of pressure in downward direction. If you are massaging these points yourself and cannot reach these points, lie back on a hard surface and position the tennis ball under the active points.

Duration: 1 min each point

48

LOCAL PAIN: *Lower Back Pain*

STEP 3: Acupressure Points B27 to B34 - *Start with a less painful side*

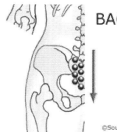

Location: on the base of the spine.

Direction: if you are massaging these points yourself and cannot reach these points, lie back on a hard surface and position the tennis ball under the active points.

Duration: 2 min

STEP 4: Acupressure Points B27 to B34 - *Switch to a more painful side*

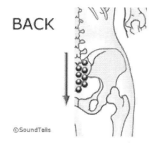

Location: on the base of the spine.

Direction: if you are massaging these points yourself and cannot reach these points, lie back on a hard surface and position the tennis ball under the active points.

Duration: 2 min

STEP 5: Acupressure Point B48 - *Start with a less painful side*

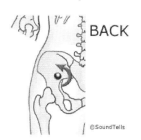

Location: in the middle of each buttock.

Direction: apply firm deep strokes of pressure in upward direction. The initial painful sensation will soon begin to subside.

Duration: 1 min

49

LOCAL PAIN: *Lower Back Pain*

STEP 6: Acupressure Point B48 - *Switch to a more painful side*

BACK

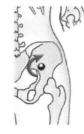

Location: in the middle of each buttock.

Direction: apply firm deep strokes of pressure in upward direction. The initial painful sensation will soon begin to subside.

Duration: 1 min

STEP 7: Acupressure Point B54 - *Start with a less painful side*

BACK

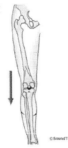

Location: in the hollow behind the knee.

Direction: apply firm deep strokes of pressure in downward direction. The initial painful sensation will soon begin to subside

Duration: 1 min

STEP 8: Acupressure Point B54 - *Switch to a more painful side*

BACK

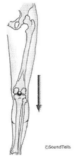

Location: in the hollow behind the knee.

Direction: apply firm deep strokes of pressure in downward direction. The initial painful sensation will soon begin to subside

Duration: 1 min

Hip Pain

Sit comfortably or lie down, close your eyes and breathe deeply when massaging the local active points.

STEP 1: Acupressure Point GB29

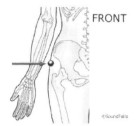

Location: on the side of the hip, in the hollow midway between the top of the hip and the top of the femur bone.

Direction: apply firm deep strokes of pressure. The initial painful sensation will soon begin to subside.

Duration: 1 min

STEP 2: Acupressure Point GB30

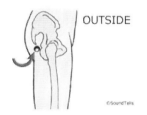

Location: in the hollow behind the top of the femur bone.

Direction: apply firm deep strokes of pressure. The initial painful sensation will soon begin to subside.

Duration: 1 min

STEP 3: Acupressure Point B48

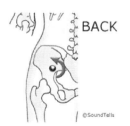

Location: in the middle of each buttock.

Direction: apply firm deep strokes of pressure in upward direction. The initial painful sensation will soon begin to subside.

Duration: 1 min

STEP 4: Acupressure Point GB34

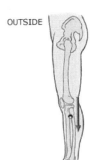

OUTSIDE

Location: bend you leg. With the tip of your index finger probe the area in front of and below the head of the outer leg bone until you feel a slight dip.

Direction: apply firm deep strokes of pressure in downward direction. The initial painful sensation will soon begin to subside.

Duration: 1 min

Knee Treatment

Acupressure is often successful in relieving knee pain. Sit comfortably or lie down, close your eyes and breathe deeply when massaging the active points.

STEP 1: Kneecap Points

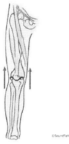

Location: in the hollow below the kneecap, on both sides of the kneecap.

Direction: apply firm deep strokes of pressure in upward direction. The initial painful sensation will soon begin to subside.

Duration: 1 min each point

STEP 2: Acupressure Point SP9

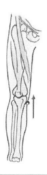

Location: on the inside of the leg, under the kneecap in the hollow just below the bulge.

Direction: apply firm deep strokes of pressure in upward direction. The initial painful sensation will soon begin to subside.

Duration: 1 min

STEP 3: Acupressure Point B54 - *Start with a less painful side*

BACK

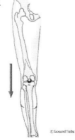

Location: in the hollow behind the knee.

Direction: apply firm deep strokes of pressure in downward direction. The initial painful sensation will soon begin to subside

Duration: 1 min

53

Ankle Treatment

Acupressure is often successful in relieving ankle pain. Sit comfortably or lie down, close your eyes and breathe deeply when massaging the local active points.

STEP 1: Acupressure Point GB40

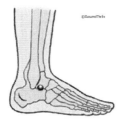

Location: in the hollow, in front of and below the outer anklebone.

Direction: apply firm deep strokes of pressure. The initial painful sensation will soon begin to subside.

Duration: 1 min

STEP 2: Acupressure Point B60

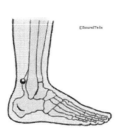

Location: in the depression between the outer anklebone and the Achilles tendon.

Direction: apply firm deep strokes of pressure. The initial painful sensation will soon begin to subside

Duration: 1 min

STEP 3: Acupressure Points K6

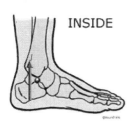

INSIDE

Location: in the depression directly below inner anklebone.

Direction: apply firm deep strokes of pressure in upward direction. The initial painful sensation will soon begin to subside

Duration: 1 min

STEP 4: Acupressure Points K3 - This point is forbidden for pregnant women

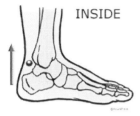 INSIDE

Location: in the hollow midway between inside anklebone and the Achilles tendon.

Direction: apply firm deep strokes of pressure in upward direction. The initial painful sensation will soon begin to subside.

Duration: 1 min

Foot Treatment

Acupressure is often successful in relieving foot pain. Sit comfortably or lie down, close your eyes and breathe deeply when massaging the local active points.

Foot Points

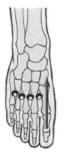 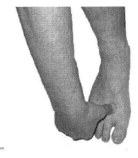

Location: on the top of the foot in the webbing between toes.

Direction: apply firm deep strokes of pressure in upward direction. The initial painful sensation will soon begin to subside.

Duration: massage every point for 2 min or until numbing feeling is produced.

Cold And Flu:
Sore Throat (tonsillitis)

Sore throat is commonly due to an infection. Acupressure is often successful in alleviating the symptoms and speeding up full recovery by improving the function of immune system. Sit comfortably or lie down, close your eyes and breathe deeply when massaging the active points.

STEP 1: Acupressure Point K27 - *Start with a less painful side*

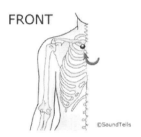

Location: in the hollow under the clavicle, next to the breastbone. To find the point follow the clavicle until it connects to the breastbone. If you have difficulty following the clavicle bone, move shoulder back and forth.

Direction: apply firm deep strokes of pressure into the chest.

Duration: 1 min

STEP 2: Acupressure Point K27 - *Switch to a more painful side*

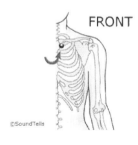

Location: in the hollow under the clavicle, next to the breastbone. To find the point follow the clavicle until it connects to the breastbone. If you have difficulty following the clavicle bone, move shoulder back and forth.

Direction: apply firm deep strokes of pressure into the chest.

Duration: 1 min

STEP 3: Acupressure Point CV22

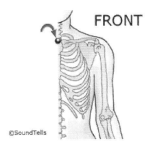

FRONT

Location: in the hollow directly below the Adam's apple.

Direction: apply firm deep strokes of pressure in downward direction. The initial painful sensation will soon begin to subside

Duration: 1 min

STEP 4: Acupressure Point Li4 - This point is forbidden for pregnant women - *Start with a less painful side*

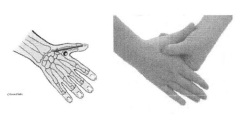

Location: between thumb and index finger as indicated on the picture.

Direction: apply firm deep strokes of pressure in upward direction. The initial painful sensation will soon begin to subside.

Duration: 2 min

STEP 5: Acupressure Point Li4 - This point is forbidden for pregnant women - *Switch to a more painful side*

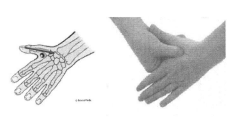

Location: between thumb and index finger as indicated on the picture.

Direction: apply firm deep strokes of pressure in upward direction. The initial painful sensation will soon begin to subside.

Duration: 2 min

STEP 6: Acupressure Point St36 - This point is forbidden for pregnant women - *Start with a less painful side*

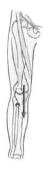

Location: with the tip of your index finger probe the area on the front side of a leg below the knee until you feel a slight dip.

Direction: apply firm deep strokes of pressure in downward direction. The initial painful sensation will soon begin to subside.

Duration: 1 min

STEP 7: Acupressure Point St36 - This point is forbidden for pregnant women - *Switch to a more painful side*

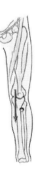

Location: with the tip of your index finger probe the area on the front side of a leg below the knee until you feel a slight dip.

Direction: apply firm deep strokes of pressure in downward direction. The initial painful sensation will soon begin to subside.

Duration: 1 min

Sinusitis (both acute and chronic)

Sinusitis is inflammation of the mucous membranes that line the inside of the nose and sinuses. Acupressure is often successful in improving the function of immune system and clearing the sinuses.

In addition to acupressure, you can use warm salt water nasal washes. Dissolve half tea spoon of table salt in a glass of warm water. Pour some solution into the palm of your hand, close one nostril, and sniff the solution into the other nostril. The saline wash should go through the nose into the mouth. Repeat several times per day.

STEP 1: Acupressure Points Li20 - *Start with a less painful side*

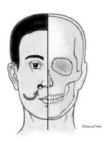

Location: in the hollow just outside each nostril.

Direction: apply firm deep strokes of pressure in upward direction. The initial painful sensation will soon begin to subside.

Duration: 1 min

STEP 2: Acupressure Point Li20 - *Switch to a more painful side*

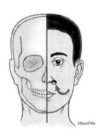

Location: in the hollow just outside each nostril.

Direction: apply firm deep strokes of pressure in upward direction. The initial painful sensation will soon begin to subside.

Duration: 1 min

STEP 3: Acupressure Point St3 - *Start with a less painful side*

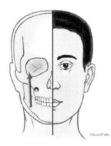

Location: below the cheekbone, directly down from the pupil of the eye.

Direction: apply firm deep strokes of pressure in upward direction against the bottom edge of the cheekbone. The initial painful sensation will soon begin to subside.

Duration: 1 min

STEP 4: Acupressure Point St3 - *Switch to a more painful side*

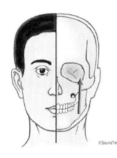

Location: below the cheekbone, directly down from the pupil of the eye.

Direction: apply firm deep strokes of pressure in upward direction against the bottom edge of the cheekbone. The initial painful sensation will soon begin to subside.

Duration: 1 min

STEP 5: Acupressure Point B2 - *Start with a less painful side*

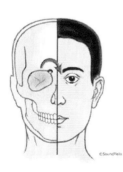

Location: with the tip of your thumb or index finger probe the area where the bridge of the nose meets the ridge of the eyebrows until you feel a slight dip.

Direction: apply firm deep strokes of pressure in downward direction. The initial painful sensation will soon begin to subside.

Duration: 1 min

STEP 6: Acupressure Point B2 - *Switch to a more painful side*

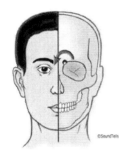

Location: with the tip of your thumb or index finger probe the area where the bridge of the nose meets the ridge of the eyebrows until you feel a slight dip.

Direction: apply firm deep strokes of pressure in downward direction. The initial painful sensation will soon begin to subside.

Duration: 1 min

STEP 7: Acupressure Point Yin Tang

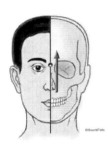

Location: with the tip of your thumb or index finger probe the area midway between the medial end of the two eyebrows as indicated on the picture until you feel a slight dip.

Direction: apply firm deep strokes of pressure in upward direction. The initial painful sensation will soon begin to subside

Duration: 1 min

STEP 8: Acupressure Point GB20 - *Start with a less painful side*

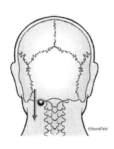

Location: just below the base of the scull, in the depression between the two major neck muscles.

Direction: apply firm deep strokes of pressure in downward direction.

Duration: 1 min

STEP 9: Acupressure Point GB20 - *Switch to a more painful side*

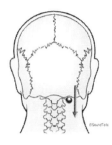

Location: just below the base of the scull, in the depression between the two major neck muscles.

Direction: apply firm deep strokes of pressure in downward direction.

Duration: 1 min

STEP 10: Acupressure Point Li4 - This point is forbidden for pregnant women - *Start with a less painful side*

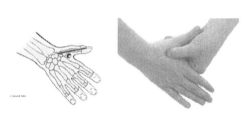

Location: between thumb and index finger as indicated on the picture.

Direction: apply firm deep strokes of pressure in upward direction. The initial painful sensation will soon begin to subside.

Duration: 2 min

STEP 11: Acupressure Point Li4 - This point is forbidden for pregnant women - *Switch to a more painful side*

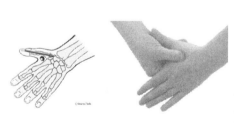

Location: between thumb and index finger as indicated on the picture.

Direction: apply firm deep strokes of pressure in upward direction. The initial painful sensation will soon begin to subside.

Duration: 2 min

Earache

The most common cause of earache is infection of the middle ear (otitis media). Most ear infections will resolve on their own. Occasionally antibiotics are prescribed to treat the infection. Acupressure speeds up recovery as well as relieves symptoms of earache. Sit comfortably or lie down, close your eyes and breathe deeply when massaging the active points.

STEP 1: Ear Point Si19, GB2, TW21 - *Start with a less painful side*

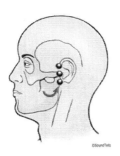

Location: Si9 is in the front of the ear hole in the hollow that becomes deeper when the mouth is open. GB2 is in the depression half finger-width below Si9. TW21 is in the depression half finger-width above Si9.

Direction: apply firm deep strokes of pressure. The initial painful sensation will soon begin to subside.

Duration: massage every point for about 1 min.

STEP 2: Ear Point Si19, GB2, TW21 - *Switch to a more painful side*

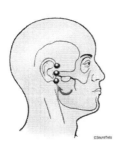

Location: Si9 is in the front of the ear hole in the hollow that becomes deeper when the mouth is open. GB2 is in the depression half finger-width below Si9. TW21 is in the depression half finger-width above Si9.

Direction: apply firm deep strokes of pressure. The initial painful sensation will soon begin to subside.

Duration: massage every point for about 1 min.

STEP 3: Acupressure Point TW17 - *Start with a less painful side*

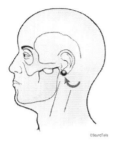

Location: in the hollow behind the ear lobe.

Direction: take a deep breath and slowly breathe out while holding this point.

Duration: 2 min

STEP 4: Acupressure Point TW17 - *Switch to a more painful side*

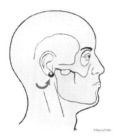

Location: in the hollow behind the ear lobe.

Direction: take a deep breath and slowly breathe out while holding this point.

Duration: 2 min

STEP 5: Acupressure Point GB20 - *Start with a less painful side*

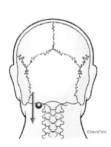

Location: just below the base of the scull, in the depression between the two major neck muscles.

Direction: apply firm deep strokes of pressure in downward direction.

Duration: 1 min

STEP 6: Acupressure Point GB20 - *Switch to a more painful side*

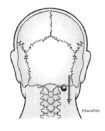

Location: just below the base of the scull, in the depression between the two major neck muscles.

Direction: apply firm deep strokes of pressure in downward direction.

Duration: 1 min

STEP 7: Acupressure Points K3 - This point is forbidden for pregnant women - *Start with a less painful side*

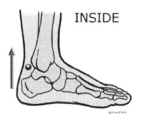

INSIDE

Location: in the hollow midway between inside anklebone and the Achilles tendon.

Direction: apply firm deep strokes of pressure in upward direction. The initial painful sensation will soon begin to subside.

Duration: 1 min

STEP 8: Acupressure Point K3 - This point is forbidden for pregnant women - *Switch to a more painful side*

INSIDE

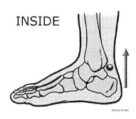

Location: in the hollow midway between inside anklebone and the Achilles tendon.

Direction: apply firm deep strokes of pressure in upward direction. The initial painful sensation will soon begin to subside.

Duration: 1 min

Loss Of Voice (laryngitis)

Loss of voice is often due to inflammation of the larynx. Acupressure is often successful in speeding up the recovery. Sit comfortably or lie down, close your eyes and breathe deeply when massaging the active points.

STEP 1: Acupressure Point CV22

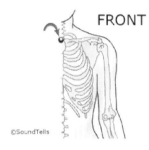

Location: in the hollow directly below the Adam's apple.

Direction: apply firm deep strokes of pressure in downward direction. The initial painful sensation will soon begin to subside

Duration: 1 min

STEP 2: Acupressure Point K27 - *Start with a less painful side*

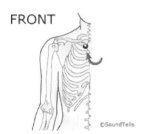

Location: in the hollow under the clavicle, next to the breastbone. To find the point follow the clavicle until it connects to the breastbone. If you have difficulty following the clavicle bone, move shoulder back and forth.

Direction: apply firm deep strokes of pressure into the chest.

Duration: 1 min

STEP 3: Acupressure Point K27 - *Switch to a more painful side*

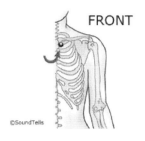

Location: in the hollow under the clavicle, next to the breastbone. To find the point follow the clavicle until it connects to the breastbone. If you have difficulty following the clavicle bone, move shoulder back and forth.

Direction: apply firm deep strokes of pressure into the chest.

Duration: 1 min

STEP 4: Acupressure Point Lu7 - *Start with a less painful side*

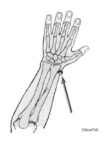

Location: on the side of the arm, one thumb-width away from the wrist crest.

Direction: apply firm deep strokes of pressure in upward direction. The initial painful sensation will soon begin to subside.

Duration: 1 min

STEP 5: Acupressure Point Lu7 - *Switch to a more painful side*

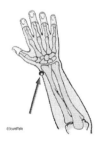

Location: on the side of the arm, one thumb-width away from the wrist crest.

Direction: apply firm deep strokes of pressure in upward direction. The initial painful sensation will soon begin to subside.

Duration: 1 min

COLD AND FLU: *Loss Of Voice*

STEP 6: Acupressure Point Li4 - This point is forbidden for pregnant women - *Start with a less painful side*

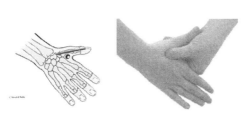

Location: between thumb and index finger as indicated on the picture.

Direction: apply firm deep strokes of pressure in upward direction. The initial painful sensation will soon begin to subside.

Duration: 2 min

STEP 7: Acupressure Point Li4 - This point is forbidden for pregnant women - *Switch to a more painful side*

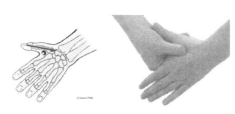

Location: between thumb and index finger as indicated on the picture.

Direction: apply firm deep strokes of pressure in upward direction. The initial painful sensation will soon begin to subside.

Duration: 2 min

69

Nervous System:
Anxiety Attacks And Nervousness

As scary as they are, periods of nervousness and occasional anxiety attacks are NORMAL. I have yet to meet a person who have never experienced these problems.

Use the combination of exercise, diet, and acupressure treatment for best results. The combination treatment has a synergistic effect that is much more pronounced than that of either treatment alone:

1. Exercise for at least 30 consecutive minutes every day - endurance exercise like running and swimming works best. Do not interrupt the exercise. After consecutive 30 minutes of exercise endorphin is released into the blood stream. Endorphin is a natural body painkiller. Endorphin and morphine are chemically different molecules but, by coincidence, they have very similar 3-dimensional shape. This similarity in shape allows morphine to bind the endorphin receptor, reduce pain, and induce feeling of euphoria. The endorphin released by exercise and acupressure treatment will improve your mood and will eventually lead to complete disappearance of anxiety.
2. Exclude caffeinated drinks such as tea, coffee, and cola from your diet until the symptoms disappear. If you cannot stop yourself from drinking tea and coffee, then switch to decaffeinated version of the drink. The decaffeination process of coffee and tea effectively removes over 90% of caffeine. Exclude chocolate.
3. Treat active points for as long as you can or until numbing feeling is produced. Repeat the treatment as often as you can during the day.

Sit comfortably or lie down, close your eyes when massaging the active points, breathe slow and deep.

70

STEP 1: Acupressure Point P6 - *Start with a less painful side*

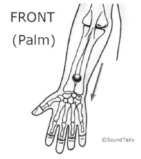

Location: on the interior side of the arm, in the hollow between the bones of the forearm, three finger-width above the wrist crease.

Direction: apply firm deep strokes of pressure in the direction of the palm. The initial painful sensation will soon begin to subside

Duration: 3 min or more

STEP 2: Acupressure Point P6 - *Switch to a more painful side*

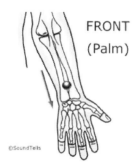

Location: on the interior side of the arm, in the hollow between the bones of the forearm, three finger-width above the wrist crease.

Direction: apply firm deep strokes of pressure in the direction of the palm. The initial painful sensation will soon begin to subside

Duration: 3 min or more

STEP 3: Acupressure Point H7 - *Start with a less painful side*

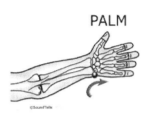

Location: on the inside of the arm; in the hollow formed by the wrist, inside bone of the arm, and the tendon. To find the point: 1. straiten the wrist; 2. slide your thumb along the wrist crease until the thumb falls into a hollow formed by the tendon, inside bone of the arm, and the wrist.

Direction: apply firm deep strokes of pressure in direction of the palm. The initial painful sensation will soon begin to subside

Duration: 1 min or more

STEP 4: Acupressure Point H7 - *Switch to a more painful side*

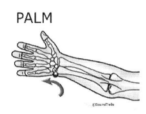

Location: on the inside of the arm; in the hollow formed by the wrist, inside bone of the arm, and the tendon. To find the point: 1. straiten the wrist; 2. slide your thumb along the wrist crease until the thumb falls into a hollow formed by the tendon, inside bone of the arm, and the wrist.

Direction: apply firm deep strokes of pressure in direction of the palm. The initial painful sensation will soon begin to subside

Duration: 1 min or more

STEP 5: Acupressure Point TW15 - *Start with a less painful side*

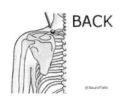

Location: on the top of the shoulder blade. To find the point go directly up from the nipple, around the top of the trapezoid muscle, and down to the top of the shoulder blade.

Direction: apply firm deep strokes of pressure in upward direction. The initial painful sensation will soon begin to subside

Duration: 1 min or more

STEP 6: Acupressure Point TW15 - *Switch to a more painful side*

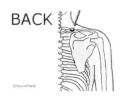

Location: on the top of the shoulder blade. To find the point go directly up from the nipple, around the top of the trapezoid muscle, and down to the top of the shoulder blade.

Direction: apply firm deep strokes of pressure in upward direction. The initial painful sensation will soon begin to subside

Duration: 1 min or more

STEP 7: Acupressure Point CV17

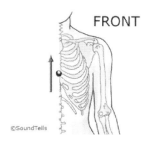

Location: in the center of the breastbone, midway between nipples.

Direction: apply firm deep strokes of pressure in upward direction. The initial painful sensation will soon begin to subside.

Duration: 2 min or more

STEP 8: Acupressure Point Yin Tang

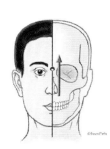

Location: with the tip of your thumb or index finger probe the area midway between the medial end of the two eyebrows as indicated on the picture until you feel a slight dip.

Direction: apply firm deep strokes of pressure in upward direction. The initial painful sensation will soon begin to subside

Duration: 1 min or more

Depression

Use the combination of exercise, diet, change in attitude, and acupressure treatment for best results. The combination has a synergistic effect that is much more pronounced than that of either treatment alone:

1. Exercise for at least 30 consecutive minutes every day. A repetitive exercise such as swimming or jogging works the best. Do not interrupt the exercise. After consecutive 30 minutes of exercise endorphin is released into the blood stream. Endorphin is a natural body painkiller. Endorphin and morphine are chemically different molecules but, by coincidence, they have very similar 3-dimensional shape. This similarity in shape allows morphine to bind the endorphin receptor, reduce pain, and induce feeling of euphoria. The endorphin released by exercise and acupressure treatment will improve your mood and will eventually lead to complete disappearance of depression.
2. In most people caffeine tends to increase nervousness and agitation. Therefore exclude tea, coffee, and other caffeinated beverages from your diet. If you absolutely cannot exclude coffee or tea, switch to decaffeinated beverages. The decaffeination process of coffee and tea effectively removes over 90% of caffeine.
3. Change your attitude – you CANNOT be guilty for everything you blame yourself.
4. Start a diary – write down a list of problems and possible solutions to each problem. If there is no solution, write no solution.
5. Treat active points for as long as you can or until numbing feeling is produced. Repeat the treatment as often as you can during the day.

When massaging active points lie comfortably in bed, close your eyes and breathe deeply. Treat active points until numbing feeling is produced.

STEP 1: Acupressure Point GV20

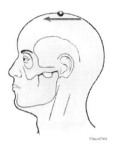

Location: with the tip of your index finger probe the area on the top of the head, where the line connecting the high points of your ears crosses the body midline until you feel a slight dip.

Direction: apply firm deep circular strokes of pressure in the forward direction. The initial painful sensation will soon begin to subside.

Duration: 2 min

STEP 2: Acupressure Point GB20 - *Start with a less painful side*

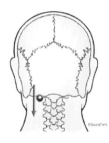

Location: just below the base of the scull, in the depression between the two major neck muscles.

Direction: apply firm deep strokes of pressure in downward direction.

Duration: 1 min

STEP 3: Acupressure Point GB20 - *Switch to a more painful side*

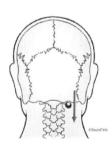

Location: just below the base of the scull, in the depression between the two major neck muscles.

Direction: apply firm deep strokes of pressure in downward direction.

Duration: 1 min

STEP 4: Acupressure Point TW15 - *Start with a less painful side*

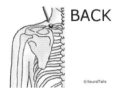

Location: on the top of the shoulder blade. To find the point go directly up from the nipple, around the top of the trapezoid muscle, and down to the top of the shoulder blade.

Direction: apply firm deep strokes of pressure in upward direction. The initial painful sensation will soon begin to subside

Duration: 1 min

STEP 5: Acupressure Point TW15 - *Switch to a more painful side*

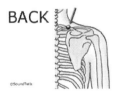

Location: on the top of the shoulder blade. To find the point go directly up from the nipple, around the top of the trapezoid muscle, and down to the top of the shoulder blade.

Direction: apply firm deep strokes of pressure in upward direction. The initial painful sensation will soon begin to subside

Duration: 1 min

STEP 6: Acupressure Point Yin Tang

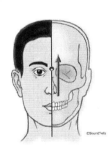

Location: with the tip of your thumb or index finger probe the area midway between the medial end of the two eyebrows as indicated on the picture until you feel a slight dip.

Direction: apply firm deep strokes of pressure in upward direction. The initial painful sensation will soon begin to subside

Duration: 1 min

STEP 7: Acupressure Point CV17

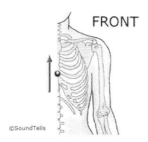

Location: in the center of the breastbone, midway between nipples.

Direction: apply firm deep strokes of pressure in upward direction. The initial painful sensation will soon begin to subside.

Duration: 2 min

STEP 8: Acupressure Point K27 - *Start with a less painful side*

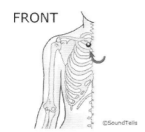

Location: in the hollow under the clavicle, next to the breastbone. To find the point follow the clavicle until it connects to the breastbone. If you have difficulty following the clavicle bone, move shoulder back and forth.

Direction: apply firm deep strokes of pressure into the chest.

Duration: 1 min

STEP 9: Acupressure Point K27 - *Switch to a more painful side*

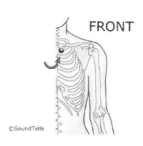

Location: in the hollow under the clavicle, next to the breastbone. To find the point follow the clavicle until it connects to the breastbone. If you have difficulty following the clavicle bone, move shoulder back and forth.

Direction: apply firm deep strokes of pressure into the chest.

Duration: 1 min

STEP 10: Acupressure Point Lu1 - *Start with a less painful side*

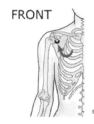

Location: on the outside edge of the rib cage, three finger-width below the clavicle.

Direction: apply firm deep strokes of pressure into the chest.

Duration: 1 min

STEP 11: Acupressure Point Lu1 - *Switch to a more painful side*

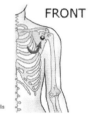

Location: on the outside edge of the rib cage, three finger-width below the clavicle.

Direction: apply firm deep strokes of pressure into the chest.

Duration: 1 min

STEP 12: Acupressure Point St36 - **This point is forbidden for pregnant women** - *Start with a less painful side*

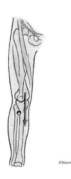

Location: with the tip of your index finger probe the area on the front side of a leg below the knee until you feel a slight dip.

Direction: apply firm deep strokes of pressure in downward direction. The initial painful sensation will soon begin to subside.

Duration: 1 min

NERVOUS SYSTEM: *Depression*

STEP 13: Acupressure Point St36 - This point is forbidden for pregnant women - *Switch to a more painful side*

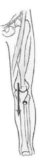

Location: with the tip of your index finger probe the area on the front side of a leg below the knee until you feel a slight dip.

Direction: apply firm deep strokes of pressure in downward direction. The initial painful sensation will soon begin to subside.

Duration: 1 min

79

Relieving Insomnia

Everyone experiences insomnia from time to time. Use combination of exercise, diet, and acupressure treatment to achieve best results. The combination has a synergistic effect that is much more pronounced than that of either treatment alone:

1. Exercise for at least 30 consecutive minutes every day. A repetitive exercise such as swimming or jogging works the best. Do not interrupt the exercise. After consecutive 30 minutes of exercise endorphin is released into the blood stream. Endorphin is a natural body painkiller. Endorphin and morphine are chemically different molecules but, by coincidence, they have very similar 3-dimensional shape. This similarity in shape allows morphine to bind the endorphin receptor, reduce pain, and induce feeling of euphoria. The endorphin released by exercise and acupressure treatment will improve your mood and will eventually lead to complete disappearance of insomnia.
2. Do not drink tea, coffee, or any other caffeinated beverages for at least 6 hours before going to bed.
3. Get up at the same time every morning. Start a day with plenty of light. Bright light resets the internal circadian clock that regulates sleep-wakefulness pattern.
4. Avoid taking naps during the day.
5. Use your bed for sleep only, not for reading during the day or TV.
6. Do not tense up at the thought that you won't get a full eight hours of sleep – occasional lack of sleep has no effect on your health. Many people including Napoleon and Churchill were able to get by on 3 to 5 hours of sleep.
7. Do not worry if you wake up in the middle of the night. Recent research indicates that humans might be genetically predisposed to biphasic sleep. Stay in bed, read a book and avoid bright light. You are very likely to fall asleep in the next 60 to 90 minutes.
8. Each night before going to bed write down everything you are thinking about on a piece of paper. Write down a list of problems and possible solutions to each problem. If there is no solution, write no solution.
9. Neither work on your PC nor watch TV for at least 30 minutes before going to bed, you may want to read a book instead.

When massaging active points lie comfortably in bed, close your eyes and breathe deeply. Cover the walls of the bedroom with Peace, Love, and Kindness. Treat active points until numbing feeling is produced or until you fall asleep. You do not need to treat all points.

NERVOUS SYSTEM: *Relieving Insomnia*

STEP 1: Acupressure Point GB20 - *Start with a less painful side*

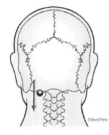

Location: just below the base of the scull, in the depression between the two major neck muscles.

Direction: apply firm deep strokes of pressure in downward direction.

Duration: 1 min or more

STEP 2: Acupressure Point GB20 - *Switch to a more painful side*

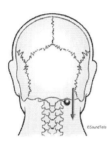

Location: just below the base of the scull, in the depression between the two major neck muscles.

Direction: apply firm deep strokes of pressure in downward direction.

Duration: 1 min or more

STEP 3: Acupressure Point GV16

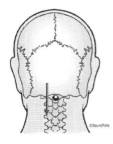

Location: in the back of the head, in the large depression under the base of the skull.

Direction: apply firm deep strokes of pressure in downward direction. The initial painful sensation will soon begin to subside.

Duration: 2 min or more

STEP 4: Acupressure Point B10 - *Start with a less painful side*

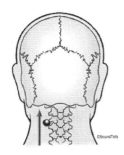

Location: halfway between the base of the skull and the base of the neck, on the edge of the trapezoid muscles.

Direction: apply firm deep strokes of pressure in upward direction. The initial painful sensation will soon begin to subside.

Duration: 1 min or more

STEP 5: Acupressure Point B10 - *Switch to a more painful side*

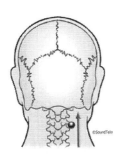

Location: halfway between the base of the skull and the base of the neck, on the edge of the trapezoid muscles.

Direction: apply firm deep strokes of pressure in upward direction. The initial painful sensation will soon begin to subside.

Duration: 1 min or more

STEP 6: Acupressure Point B38 - *Start with a less painful side*

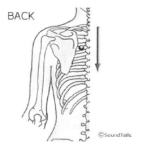

Location: four finger's width out from the spine, half way between the top and bottom of the shoulder blade, between the 4th and 5th ribs.

Direction: if you have difficulty reaching this point lie back on a hard surface and position the tennis ball under the active point. Apply firm deep strokes of pressure in downward direction. The initial painful sensation will soon begin to subside.

Duration: 1 min or more

STEP 7: Acupressure Point B38 - *Switch to a more painful side*

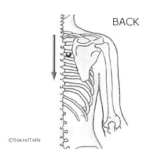

Location: four finger's width out from the spine, half way between the top and bottom of the shoulder blade, between the 4th and 5th ribs.

Direction: if you have difficulty reaching this point lie back on a hard surface and position the tennis ball under the active point. Apply firm deep strokes of pressure in downward direction. The initial painful sensation will soon begin to subside.

Duration: 1 min or more

STEP 8: Acupressure Point H7 - *Start with a less painful side*

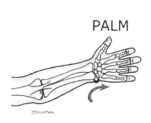

Location: on the inside of the arm; in the hollow formed by the wrist, inside bone of the arm, and the tendon. To find the point: 1. straiten the wrist; 2. slide your thumb along the wrist crease until the thumb falls into a hollow formed by the tendon, inside bone of the arm, and the wrist.

Direction: apply firm deep strokes of pressure in direction of the palm.

Duration: 1 min or more

STEP 9: Acupressure Point H7 - *Switch to a more painful side*

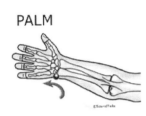

PALM

Location: on the inside of the arm; in the hollow formed by the wrist, inside bone of the arm, and the tendon. To find the point:
1. straiten the wrist; 2. slide your thumb along the wrist crease until the thumb falls into a hollow formed by the tendon, inside bone of the arm, and the wrist.

Direction: apply firm deep strokes of pressure in direction of the palm. The initial painful sensation will soon begin to subside

Duration: 1 min or more

STEP 10: Acupressure Point SP6 - This point is forbidden for pregnant women - *Start with a less painful side*

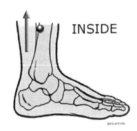

INSIDE

Location: on the inside surface of the leg, four fingers-width above the inner anklebone.

Direction: apply firm deep strokes of pressure in upward direction. The initial painful sensation will soon begin to subside

Duration: 1 min or more

STEP 11: Acupressure Point SP6 - This point is forbidden for pregnant women - *Switch to a more painful side*

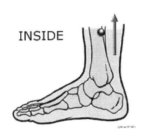

INSIDE

Location: on the inside surface of the leg, four fingers-width above the inner anklebone.

Direction: apply firm deep strokes of pressure in upward direction. The initial painful sensation will soon begin to subside

Duration: 1 min or more

STEP 12: Acupressure Points K6 - *Start with a less painful side*

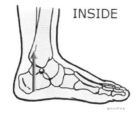

Location: in the depression directly below inner anklebone.

Direction: apply firm deep strokes of pressure in upward direction. The initial painful sensation will soon begin to subside

Duration: 1 min or more

STEP 13: Acupressure Points K6 - *Switch to a more painful side*

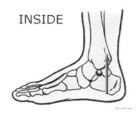

Location: in the depression directly below inner anklebone.

Direction: apply firm deep strokes of pressure in upward direction. The initial painful sensation will soon begin to subside

Duration: 1 min or more

STEP 14: Acupressure Points K3 - This point is forbidden for pregnant women - *Start with a less painful side*

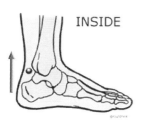

Location: in the hollow midway between inside anklebone and the Achilles tendon.

Direction: apply firm deep strokes of pressure in upward direction. The initial painful sensation will soon begin to subside.

Duration: 1 min

STEP 15: Acupressure Point K3 - This point is forbidden for pregnant women - *Switch to a more painful side*

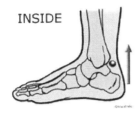

INSIDE

Location: in the hollow midway between inside anklebone and the Achilles tendon.

Direction: apply firm deep strokes of pressure in upward direction. The initial painful sensation will soon begin to subside.

Duration: 1 min

STEP 16: Acupressure Point CV17

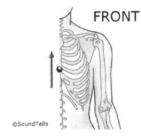

FRONT

Location: in the center of the breastbone, midway between nipples.

Direction: apply firm deep strokes of pressure in upward direction. The initial painful sensation will soon begin to subside.

Duration: 2 min or more

STEP 17: Acupressure Point Yin Tang

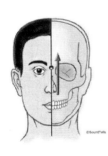

Location: with the tip of your thumb or index finger probe the area midway between the medial end of the two eyebrows as indicated on the picture until you feel a slight dip.

Direction: apply firm deep strokes of pressure in upward direction. The initial painful sensation will soon begin to subside

Duration: 1 min or more

Fainting

Avoid situations that provoke fainting. For example, you may need to eat regularly to avoid low blood sugar. You may need to get up from a bed very gradually to give vascular system enough time to adjust the blood pressure. You may need to learn to control the breathing to avoid hyperventilation when you feel worried.

Start treatment as soon as first warning signs such as dizziness, nausea, and sweaty palms appear. Sit comfortably or lie down, close your eyes and breathe deeply when massaging the active points.

STEP 1: Acupressure Point GV26

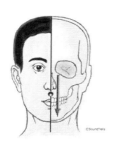

Location: in the hollow between the upper lip and the nose.

Direction: apply firm deep strokes of pressure in downward direction. The initial painful sensation will soon begin to subside.

Duration: this is the most effective active point. Massage it for 3 min or until numbing feeling is produced.

STEP 2: Acupressure Point P6 - *Start with a less painful side*

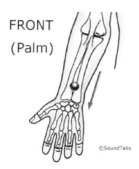

FRONT
(Palm)

Location: on the interior side of the arm, in the hollow between the bones of the forearm, three finger-width above the wrist crease.

Direction: apply firm deep strokes of pressure in the direction of the palm. The initial painful sensation will soon begin to subside

Duration: 3 min or more

STEP 3: Acupressure Point P6 - *Switch to a more painful side*

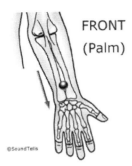

FRONT
(Palm)

Location: on the interior side of the arm, in the hollow between the bones of the forearm, three finger-width above the wrist crease.

Direction: apply firm deep strokes of pressure in the direction of the palm. The initial painful sensation will soon begin to subside

Duration: 3 min or more

STEP 4: Acupressure Point H7 - *Start with a less painful side*

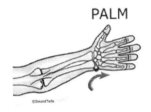

PALM

Location: on the inside of the arm; in the hollow formed by the wrist, inside bone of the arm, and the tendon. To find the point: 1. straiten the wrist; 2. slide your thumb along the wrist crease until the thumb falls into a hollow formed by the tendon, inside bone of the arm, and the wrist.

Direction: apply firm deep strokes of pressure in direction of the palm. The initial painful sensation will soon begin to subside

Duration: 1 min

STEP 5: Acupressure Point H7 - *Switch to a more painful side*

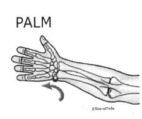

PALM

Location: on the inside of the arm; in the hollow formed by the wrist, inside bone of the arm, and the tendon. To find the point: 1. straiten the wrist; 2. slide your thumb along the wrist crease until the thumb falls into a hollow formed by the tendon, inside bone of the arm, and the wrist.

Direction: apply firm deep strokes of pressure in direction of the palm. The initial painful sensation will soon begin to subside

Duration: 1 min

STEP 6: Acupressure Point K1 - *Start with a less painful side*

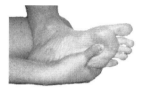

Location: in the center of the sole of the foot in the depression between the two pads.

Direction: if you are massaging this point yourself and cannot reach it, stand up with one foot on a tennis ball. Apply firm deep strokes of pressure in upward direction.

Duration: 1 min

STEP 7: Acupressure Point K1 - *Switch to a more painful side*

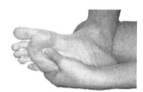

Location: in the center of the sole of the foot in the depression between the two pads.

Direction: if you are massaging this point yourself and cannot reach it, stand up with one foot on a tennis ball. Apply firm deep strokes of pressure in upward direction.

Duration: 1 min

Hiccoughs

Sit comfortably or lie down, close your eyes and breathe deeply when massaging the active points. Also close your nose and drink a glass of water with no interruption (in order to hold the breath).

STEP 1: Acupressure Point TW17 - *Start with a less painful side*

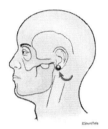

Location: in the hollow behind the ear lobe.

Direction: take a deep breath and slowly breathe out while holding this point.

Duration: 2 min

STEP 2: Acupressure Point TW17 - *Switch to a more painful side*

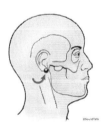

Location: in the hollow behind the ear lobe.

Direction: take a deep breath and slowly breathe out while holding this point.

Duration: 2 min

STEP 3: Acupressure Point CV22

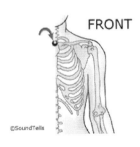

FRONT

Location: in the hollow directly below the Adam's apple.

Direction: apply firm deep strokes of pressure in downward direction. The initial painful sensation will soon begin to subside

Duration: 1 min

STEP 4: Acupressure Point CV17

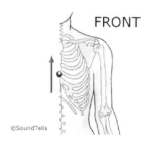

Location: in the center of the breastbone, midway between nipples.

Direction: apply firm deep strokes of pressure in upward direction. The initial painful sensation will soon begin to subside.

Duration: 2 min

STEP 5: Acupressure Point CV12

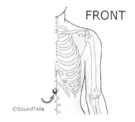

Location: midway between the belly button and the bottom of the breastbone.

Direction: apply firm deep strokes of pressure into the abdomen.

Duration: 2 min

STEP 6: Acupressure Point St36 - This point is forbidden for pregnant women - *Start with a less painful side*

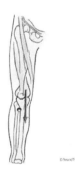

Location: with the tip of your index finger probe the area on the front side of a leg below the knee until you feel a slight dip.

Direction: apply firm deep strokes of pressure in downward direction. The initial painful sensation will soon begin to subside.

Duration: 1 min

STEP 7: Acupressure Point St36 - This point is forbidden for pregnant women - *Switch to a more painful side*

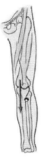

Location: with the tip of your index finger probe the area on the front side of a leg below the knee until you feel a slight dip.

Direction: apply firm deep strokes of pressure in downward direction. The initial painful sensation will soon begin to subside.

Duration: 1 min

Memory And Concentration Improvement

Sit comfortably or lie down, close your eyes and breathe deeply when massaging the active points.

STEP 1: Acupressure Point TW15 - *Start with a less painful side*

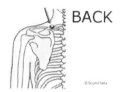

Location: on the top of the shoulder blade. To find the point go directly up from the nipple, around the top of the trapezoid muscle, and down to the top of the shoulder blade.

Direction: apply firm deep strokes of pressure in upward direction. The initial painful sensation will soon begin to subside

Duration: 1 min

STEP 2: Acupressure Point TW15 - *Switch to a more painful side*

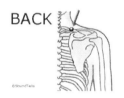

Location: on the top of the shoulder blade. To find the point go directly up from the nipple, around the top of the trapezoid muscle, and down to the top of the shoulder blade.

Direction: apply firm deep strokes of pressure in upward direction. The initial painful sensation will soon begin to subside

Duration: 1 min

STEP 3: Acupressure Point GB20 - *Start with a less painful side*

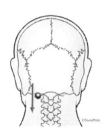

Location: just below the base of the scull, in the depression between the two major neck muscles.

Direction: apply firm deep strokes of pressure in downward direction.

Duration: 1 min

STEP 4: Acupressure Point GB20 - *Switch to a more painful side*

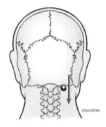

Location: just below the base of the scull, in the depression between the two major neck muscles.

Direction: apply firm deep strokes of pressure in downward direction.

Duration: 1 min

STEP 5: Acupressure Point Yin Tang

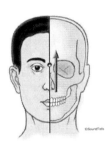

Location: with the tip of your thumb or index finger probe the area midway between the medial end of the two eyebrows as indicated on the picture until you feel a slight dip.

Direction: apply firm deep strokes of pressure in upward direction. The initial painful sensation will soon begin to subside

Duration: 1 min

STEP 6: Acupressure Point GV26

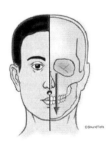

Location: in the hollow between the upper lip and the nose.

Direction: apply firm deep strokes of pressure in downward direction. The initial painful sensation will soon begin to subside.

Duration: 1 min

STEP 7: Acupressure Point CV17

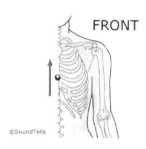
FRONT
©SoundTells

Location: in the center of the breastbone, midway between nipples.

Direction: apply firm deep strokes of pressure in upward direction. The initial painful sensation will soon begin to subside.

Duration: 2 min

Cardiovascular System:
Angina Treatment

Acupressure offers only symptomatic relief to angina and palpitations. Patients with these conditions should seek a qualified medical advice.

STEP 1: Acupressure Point CV17

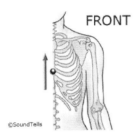

Location: in the center of the breastbone, midway between nipples.

Direction: apply firm deep strokes of pressure in upward direction. The initial painful sensation will soon begin to subside.

Duration: 2 min

STEP 2: Acupressure Point P6 - *Start with a less painful side*

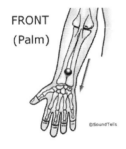

Location: on the interior side of the arm, in the hollow between the bones of the forearm, three finger-width above the wrist crease.

Direction: apply firm deep strokes of pressure in the direction of the palm. The initial painful sensation will soon begin to subside

Duration: 3 min or more

STEP 3: Acupressure Point P6 - *Switch to a more painful side*

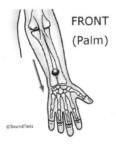

Location: on the interior side of the arm, in the hollow between the bones of the forearm, three finger-width above the wrist crease.

Direction: apply firm deep strokes of pressure in the direction of the palm. The initial painful sensation will soon begin to subside

Duration: 3 min or more

STEP 4: Acupressure Point H7 - *Start with a less painful side*

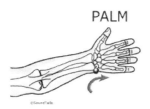

PALM

Location: on the inside of the arm; in the hollow formed by the wrist, inside bone of the arm, and the tendon. To find the point: 1. straiten the wrist; 2. slide your thumb along the wrist crease until the thumb falls into a hollow formed by the tendon, inside bone of the arm, and the wrist.

Direction: apply firm deep strokes of pressure in direction of the palm. The initial painful sensation will soon begin to subside

Duration: 1 min

STEP 5: Acupressure Point H7 - *Switch to a more painful side*

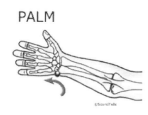

PALM

Location: on the inside of the arm; in the hollow formed by the wrist, inside bone of the arm, and the tendon. To find the point: 1. straiten the wrist; 2. slide your thumb along the wrist crease until the thumb falls into a hollow formed by the tendon, inside bone of the arm, and the wrist.

Direction: apply firm deep strokes of pressure in direction of the palm. The initial painful sensation will soon begin to subside

Duration: 1 min

STEP 6: Acupressure Point Yin Tang

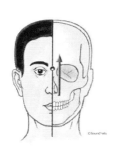

Location: with the tip of your thumb or index finger probe the area midway between the medial end of the two eyebrows as indicated on the picture until you feel a slight dip.

Direction: apply firm deep strokes of pressure in upward direction. The initial painful sensation will soon begin to subside

Duration: 1 min

Palpitations Treatment

Acupressure offers only symptomatic relief to angina and palpitations. Patients with these conditions should seek a qualified medical advice.

Sit comfortably or lie down, close your eyes and breathe deeply when massaging the active points.

STEP 1: Acupressure Point P6 - *Start with a less painful side*

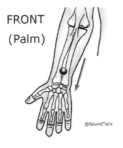

Location: on the interior side of the arm, in the hollow between the bones of the forearm, three finger-width above the wrist crease.

Direction: apply firm deep strokes of pressure in the direction of the palm. The initial painful sensation will soon begin to subside

Duration: 3 min or more

STEP 2: Acupressure Point P6 - *Switch to a more painful side*

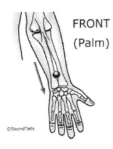

Location: on the interior side of the arm, in the hollow between the bones of the forearm, three finger-width above the wrist crease.

Direction: apply firm deep strokes of pressure in the direction of the palm. The initial painful sensation will soon begin to subside

Duration: 3 min or more

STEP 3: Acupressure Point H7 - *Start with a less painful side*

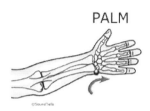

PALM

Location: on the inside of the arm; in the hollow formed by the wrist, inside bone of the arm, and the tendon. To find the point: 1. straiten the wrist; 2. slide your thumb along the wrist crease until the thumb falls into a hollow formed by the tendon, inside bone of the arm, and the wrist.

Direction: apply firm deep strokes of pressure in direction of the palm. The initial painful sensation will soon begin to subside

Duration: 1 min

STEP 4: Acupressure Point H7 - *Switch to a more painful side*

PALM

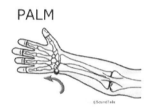

Location: on the inside of the arm; in the hollow formed by the wrist, inside bone of the arm, and the tendon. To find the point: 1. straiten the wrist; 2. slide your thumb along the wrist crease until the thumb falls into a hollow formed by the tendon, inside bone of the arm, and the wrist.

Direction: apply firm deep strokes of pressure in direction of the palm. The initial painful sensation will soon begin to subside

Duration: 1 min

STEP 5: Acupressure Point Yin Tang

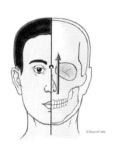

Location: with the tip of your thumb or index finger probe the area midway between the medial end of the two eyebrows as indicated on the picture until you feel a slight dip.

Direction: apply firm deep strokes of pressure in upward direction. The initial painful sensation will soon begin to subside

Duration: 1 min

STEP 6: Acupressure Point TW15 - *Start with a less painful side*

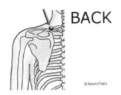

Location: on the top of the shoulder blade. To find the point go directly up from the nipple, around the top of the trapezoid muscle, and down to the top of the shoulder blade.

Direction: apply firm deep strokes of pressure in upward direction. The initial painful sensation will soon begin to subside

Duration: 1 min

STEP 7: Acupressure Point TW15 - *Switch to a more painful side*

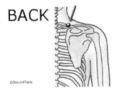

Location: on the top of the shoulder blade. To find the point go directly up from the nipple, around the top of the trapezoid muscle, and down to the top of the shoulder blade.

Direction: apply firm deep strokes of pressure in upward direction. The initial painful sensation will soon begin to subside

Duration: 1 min

High Blood Pressure Treatment

High blood pressure is a common condition. Acupressure is often an effective method to control high blood pressure. Sit comfortably or lie down, close your eyes and breathe deeply when massaging the active points.

STEP 1: Acupressure Point P6 - *Start with a less painful side*

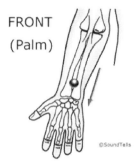

FRONT
(Palm)

Location: on the interior side of the arm, in the hollow between the bones of the forearm, three finger-width above the wrist crease.

Direction: apply firm deep strokes of pressure in the direction of the palm. The initial painful sensation will soon begin to subside

Duration: 3 min or more

STEP 2: Acupressure Point P6 - *Switch to a more painful side*

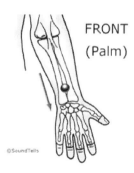

FRONT
(Palm)

Location: on the interior side of the arm, in the hollow between the bones of the forearm, three finger-width above the wrist crease.

Direction: apply firm deep strokes of pressure in the direction of the palm. The initial painful sensation will soon begin to subside

Duration: 3 min or more

STEP 3: Acupressure Point St36 - This point is forbidden for pregnant women - *Start with a less painful side*

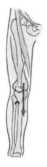

Location: with the tip of your index finger probe the area on the front side of a leg below the knee until you feel a slight dip.

Direction: apply firm deep strokes of pressure in downward direction. The initial painful sensation will soon begin to subside.

Duration: 1 min

STEP 4: Acupressure Point St36 - This point is forbidden for pregnant women - *Switch to a more painful side*

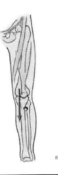

Location: with the tip of your index finger probe the area on the front side of a leg below the knee until you feel a slight dip.

Direction: apply firm deep strokes of pressure in downward direction. The initial painful sensation will soon begin to subside.

Duration: 1 min

STEP 5: Acupressure Points K3 - This point is forbidden for pregnant women - *Start with a less painful side*

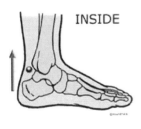

INSIDE

Location: in the hollow midway between inside anklebone and the Achilles tendon.

Direction: apply firm deep strokes of pressure in upward direction. The initial painful sensation will soon begin to subside.

Duration: 1 min

STEP 6: Acupressure Point K3 - This point is forbidden for pregnant women - *Switch to a more painful side*

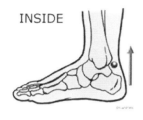

INSIDE

Location: in the hollow midway between inside anklebone and the Achilles tendon.

Direction: apply firm deep strokes of pressure in upward direction. The initial painful sensation will soon begin to subside.

Duration: 1 min

STEP 7: Acupressure Point TW15 - *Start with a less painful side*

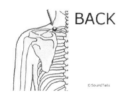

BACK

Location: on the top of the shoulder blade. To find the point go directly up from the nipple, around the top of the trapezoid muscle, and down to the top of the shoulder blade.

Direction: apply firm deep strokes of pressure in upward direction. The initial painful sensation will soon begin to subside

Duration: 1 min

STEP 8: Acupressure Point TW15 - *Switch to a more painful side*

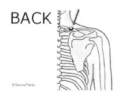

BACK

Location: on the top of the shoulder blade. To find the point go directly up from the nipple, around the top of the trapezoid muscle, and down to the top of the shoulder blade.

Direction: apply firm deep strokes of pressure in upward direction. The initial painful sensation will soon begin to subside

Duration: 1 min

Abdominal Discomfort:
Constipation

Sit comfortably or lie down, close your eyes and breathe deeply when massaging the active points.

STEP 1: Acupressure Point SP15 - *Start with a less painful side*

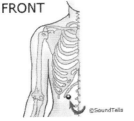

Location: on the intersection of nipple line and belly button line.

Direction: apply firm deep strokes of pressure into the abdomen. The initial painful sensation will soon begin to subside

Duration: 1 min

STEP 2: Acupressure Point SP15 - *Switch to a more painful side*

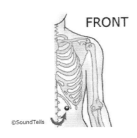

Location: on the intersection of nipple line and belly button line.

Direction: apply firm deep strokes of pressure into the abdomen. The initial painful sensation will soon begin to subside

Duration: 1 min

STEP 3: Acupressure Point CV6

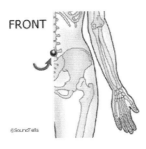

Location: two fingers-width below the belly button.

Direction: apply firm deep strokes of pressure into the abdomen. The initial painful sensation will soon begin to subside.

Duration: 1 min

STEP 4: Acupressure Point Li4 - This point is forbidden for pregnant women - *Start with a less painful side*

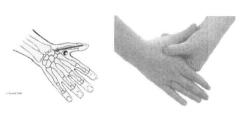

Location: between thumb and index finger as indicated on the picture.

Direction: apply firm deep strokes of pressure in upward direction. The initial painful sensation will soon begin to subside.

Duration: 2 min

STEP 5: Acupressure Point Li4 - This point is forbidden for pregnant women - *Switch to a more painful side*

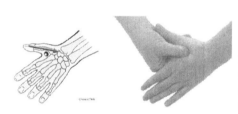

Location: between thumb and index finger as indicated on the picture.

Direction: apply firm deep strokes of pressure in upward direction. The initial painful sensation will soon begin to subside.

Duration: 2 min

STEP 6: Acupressure Point St36 - This point is forbidden for pregnant women - *Start with a less painful side*

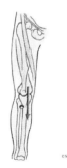

Location: with the tip of your index finger probe the area on the front side of a leg below the knee until you feel a slight dip.

Direction: apply firm deep strokes of pressure in downward direction. The initial painful sensation will soon begin to subside.

Duration: 1 min

STEP 7: Acupressure Point St36 - This point is forbidden for pregnant women - *Switch to a more painful side*

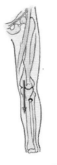

Location: with the tip of your index finger probe the area on the front side of a leg below the knee until you feel a slight dip.

Direction: apply firm deep strokes of pressure in downward direction. The initial painful sensation will soon begin to subside.

Duration: 1 min

STEP 8: Acupressure Point Liv3 - *Start with a less painful side*

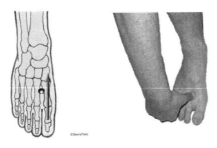

Location: on the top of the foot in the webbing between the big toe and the second toe.

Direction: apply firm deep strokes of pressure in upward direction. The initial painful sensation will soon begin to subside.

Duration: 1 min

STEP 9: Acupressure Point Liv3 - *Switch to a more painful side*

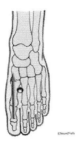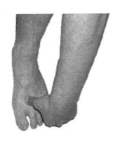

Location: on the top of the foot in the webbing between the big toe and the second toe.

Direction: apply firm deep strokes of pressure in upward direction. The initial painful sensation will soon begin to subside.

Duration: 1 min

Diarrhea

Sit comfortably or lie down, close your eyes and breathe deeply when massaging the active points.

STEP 1: Acupressure Point SP15 - *Start with a less painful side*

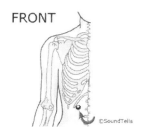

Location: on the intersection of nipple line and belly button line.

Direction: apply firm deep strokes of pressure into the abdomen. The initial painful sensation will soon begin to subside

Duration: 1 min

STEP 2: Acupressure Point SP15 - *Switch to a more painful side*

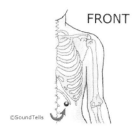

Location: on the intersection of nipple line and belly button line.

Direction: apply firm deep strokes of pressure into the abdomen. The initial painful sensation will soon begin to subside

Duration: 1 min

STEP 3: Acupressure Point CV6

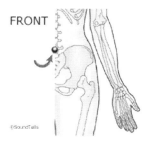

Location: two fingers-width below the belly button.

Direction: apply firm deep strokes of pressure into the abdomen. The initial painful sensation will soon begin to subside.

Duration: 1 min

STEP 4: Acupressure Point Li4 - This point is forbidden for pregnant women - *Start with a less painful side*

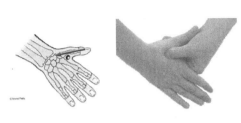

Location: between thumb and index finger as indicated on the picture.

Direction: apply firm deep strokes of pressure in upward direction. The initial painful sensation will soon begin to subside.

Duration: 2 min

STEP 5: Acupressure Point Li4 - This point is forbidden for pregnant women - *Switch to a more painful side*

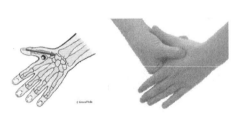

Location: between thumb and index finger as indicated on the picture.

Direction: apply firm deep strokes of pressure in upward direction. The initial painful sensation will soon begin to subside.

Duration: 2 min

STEP 6: Acupressure Point St36 - This point is forbidden for pregnant women - *Start with a less painful side*

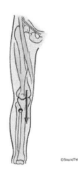

Location: with the tip of your index finger probe the area on the front side of a leg below the knee until you feel a slight dip.

Direction: apply firm deep strokes of pressure in downward direction. The initial painful sensation will soon begin to subside.

Duration: 1 min

STEP 7: Acupressure Point St36 - This point is forbidden for pregnant women - *Switch to a more painful side*

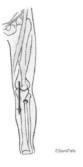

Location: with the tip of your index finger probe the area on the front side of a leg below the knee until you feel a slight dip.

Direction: apply firm deep strokes of pressure in downward direction. The initial painful sensation will soon begin to subside.

Duration: 1 min

STEP 8: Acupressure Point SP4 - *Start with a less painful side*

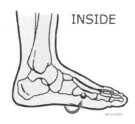

INSIDE

Location: on the arch of the foot, in the hollow two finger-width away from the ball of the foot, above the tendon of the big toe (move the big toe up and down to feel the tendon).

Direction: apply firm deep strokes of pressure in upward direction. The initial painful sensation will soon begin to subside.

Duration: 1 min

STEP 9: Acupressure Point SP4 - *Switch to a more painful side*

INSIDE

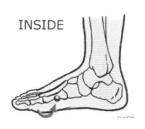

Location: on the arch of the foot, in the hollow two finger-width away from the ball of the foot, above the tendon of the big toe (move the big toe up and down to feel the tendon).

Direction: apply firm deep strokes of pressure in upward direction. The initial painful sensation will soon begin to subside.

Duration: 1 min

STEP 10: Acupressure Point Liv3 - *Start with a less painful side*

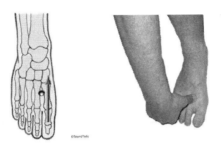

Location: on the top of the foot in the webbing between the big toe and the second toe.

Direction: apply firm deep strokes of pressure in upward direction. The initial painful sensation will soon begin to subside.

Duration: 1 min

STEP 11: Acupressure Point Liv3 - *Switch to a more painful side*

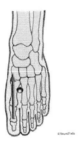
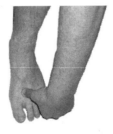

Location: on the top of the foot in the webbing between the big toe and the second toe.

Direction: apply firm deep strokes of pressure in upward direction. The initial painful sensation will soon begin to subside.

Duration: 1 min

Heartburn And Stomachache

People with heartburns and stomachaches should pay attention to their diet. As a rule of thumb avoid sweets and sweet drink and eat lots of raw vegetables and fruits. Note which particular food triggers the problem and avoid this food in the future.

Sit comfortably or lie down, close your eyes and breathe deeply when massaging the active points.

STEP 1: Acupressure Point CV12

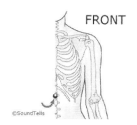

Location: midway between the belly button and the bottom of the breastbone.

Direction: apply firm deep strokes of pressure into the abdomen.

Duration: 2 min

STEP 2: Acupressure Point CV6

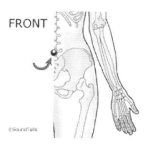

Location: two fingers-width below the belly button.

Direction: apply firm deep strokes of pressure into the abdomen. The initial painful sensation will soon begin to subside.

Duration: 1 min

ABDOMINAL: *Heartburn And Stomachache*

STEP 3: Acupressure Point P6 - *Start with a less painful side*

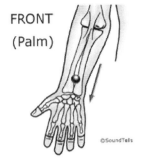

FRONT
(Palm)

Location: on the interior side of the arm, in the hollow between the bones of the forearm, three finger-width above the wrist crease.

Direction: apply firm deep strokes of pressure in the direction of the palm. The initial painful sensation will soon begin to subside

Duration: 3 min or more

STEP 4: Acupressure Point P6 - *Switch to a more painful side*

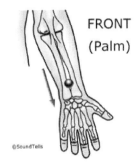

FRONT
(Palm)

Location: on the interior side of the arm, in the hollow between the bones of the forearm, three finger-width above the wrist crease.

Direction: apply firm deep strokes of pressure in the direction of the palm. The initial painful sensation will soon begin to subside

Duration: 3 min or more

STEP 5: Acupressure Point St36 - **This point is forbidden for pregnant women** - *Start with a less painful side*

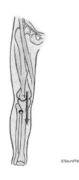

Location: with the tip of your index finger probe the area on the front side of a leg below the knee until you feel a slight dip.

Direction: apply firm deep strokes of pressure in downward direction. The initial painful sensation will soon begin to subside.

Duration: 1 min

STEP 6: Acupressure Point St36 - This point is forbidden for pregnant women - *Switch to a more painful side*

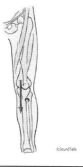

Location: with the tip of your index finger probe the area on the front side of a leg below the knee until you feel a slight dip.

Direction: apply firm deep strokes of pressure in downward direction. The initial painful sensation will soon begin to subside.

Duration: 1 min

STEP 7: Acupressure Point SP4 - *Start with a less painful side*

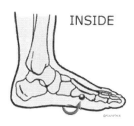

INSIDE

Location: on the arch of the foot, in the hollow two finger-width away from the ball of the foot, above the tendon of the big toe (move the big toe up and down to feel the tendon).

Direction: apply firm deep strokes of pressure in upward direction. The initial painful sensation will soon begin to subside.

Duration: 1 min

STEP 8: Acupressure Point SP4 - *Switch to a more painful side*

INSIDE

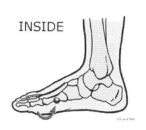

Location: on the arch of the foot, in the hollow two finger-width away from the ball of the foot, above the tendon of the big toe (move the big toe up and down to feel the tendon).

Direction: apply firm deep strokes of pressure in upward direction. The initial painful sensation will soon begin to subside.

Duration: 1 min

Women Only:
PMS And Painful Periods

PMS is due to hormonal imbalance that may start as early as two weeks before menstruation (at the time of ovulation). Acupressure is often successful in alleviating PMS symptoms. Sit comfortably or lie down, close your eyes and breathe deeply when massaging the active points.

STEP 1: Acupressure Point CV6

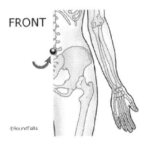

Location: two fingers-width below the belly button.

Direction: apply firm deep strokes of pressure into the abdomen. The initial painful sensation will soon begin to subside.

Duration: 1 min

STEP 2: Points SP12 and SP13 - *Start with a less painful side*

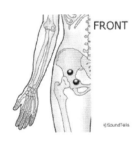

Location: **SP13** (top) in the middle of the crease where leg joins the body (groin line), one finger-width up from the top of the pubic bone, four finger-width out of the midline.
SP12 (bottom) in the middle of the crease where leg joins the body (groin line), on the top of the pubic bone, three finger-width out of the midline.

Direction: apply firm deep pressure. The initial painful sensation will soon begin to subside.

Duration: 2 min each point.

STEP 3: Points SP12 and SP13 - *Switch to a more painful side*

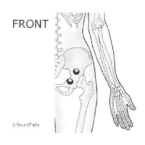

FRONT

Location: **SP13** (top) in the middle of the crease where leg joins the body (groin line), one finger-width up from the top of the pubic bone, four finger-width out of the midline.
SP12 (bottom) in the middle of the crease where leg joins the body (groin line), on the top of the pubic bone, three finger-width out of the midline.

Direction: apply firm deep pressure. The initial painful sensation will soon begin to subside.

Duration: 2 min each point.

STEP 4: Acupressure Points B27 to B34 - *Start with a less painful side*

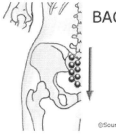

BACK **Location:** on the base of the spine.

Direction: if you are massaging these points yourself and cannot reach these points, lay back on a hard surface and position the tennis ball under the active points.

Duration: 2 min

STEP 5: Acupressure Points B27 to B34 - *Switch to a more painful side*

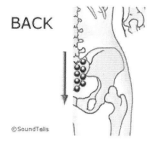

BACK **Location:** on the base of the spine.

Direction: if you are massaging these points yourself and cannot reach these points, lay back on a hard surface and position the tennis ball under the active points.

Duration: 2 min

STEP 6: Acupressure Point B48 - *Start with a less painful side*

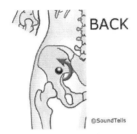

Location: in the middle of each buttock.

Direction: apply firm deep strokes of pressure in upward direction. The initial painful sensation will soon begin to subside.

Duration: 1 min

STEP 7: Acupressure Point B48 - *Switch to a more painful side*

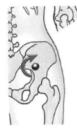

Location: in the middle of each buttock.

Direction: apply firm deep strokes of pressure in upward direction. The initial painful sensation will soon begin to subside.

Duration: 1 min

STEP 8: Acupressure Point St36 - **This point is forbidden for pregnant women** - *Start with a less painful side*

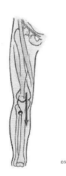

Location: with the tip of your index finger probe the area on the front side of a leg below the knee until you feel a slight dip.

Direction: apply firm deep strokes of pressure in downward direction. The initial painful sensation will soon begin to subside.

Duration: 1 min

STEP 9: Acupressure Point St36 - This point is forbidden for pregnant women - *Switch to a more painful side*

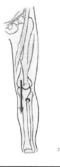

Location: with the tip of your index finger probe the area on the front side of a leg below the knee until you feel a slight dip.

Direction: apply firm deep strokes of pressure in downward direction. The initial painful sensation will soon begin to subside.

Duration: 1 min

STEP 10: Acupressure Point SP6 - This point is forbidden for pregnant women - *Start with a less painful side*

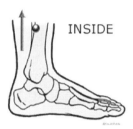

INSIDE

Location: on the inside surface of the leg, four fingers-width above the inner anklebone.

Direction: apply firm deep strokes of pressure in upward direction. The initial painful sensation will soon begin to subside

Duration: 1 min

STEP 11: Acupressure Point SP6 - This point is forbidden for pregnant women - *Switch to a more painful side*

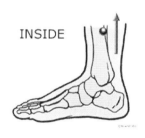

INSIDE

Location: on the inside surface of the leg, four fingers-width above the inner anklebone.

Direction: apply firm deep strokes of pressure in upward direction. The initial painful sensation will soon begin to subside

Duration: 1 min

WOMEN ONLY: *PMS And Painful Periods*

STEP 12: Acupressure Point Liv3 - *Start with a less painful side*

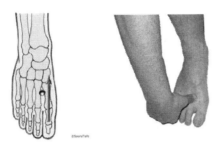

Location: on the top of the foot in the webbing between the big toe and the second toe.

Direction: apply firm deep strokes of pressure in upward direction. The initial painful sensation will soon begin to subside.

Duration: 1 min

STEP 13: Acupressure Point Liv3 - *Switch to a more painful side*

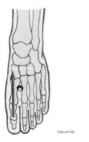 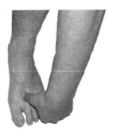

Location: on the top of the foot in the webbing between the big toe and the second toe.

Direction: apply firm deep strokes of pressure in upward direction. The initial painful sensation will soon begin to subside.

Duration: 1 min

Hot Flashes

Hot flashes are normal part of going through menopause. They are due to hormonal imbalance that occur at this time. Regular acupressure treatments, even when no hot flashes are occurring, are most helpful. Sit comfortably or lie down, close your eyes and breathe deeply when massaging the active points.

STEP 1: Acupressure Point CV17

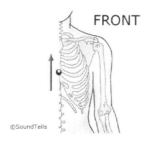

Location: in the center of the breastbone, midway between nipples.

Direction: apply firm deep strokes of pressure in upward direction. The initial painful sensation will soon begin to subside.

Duration: 2 min

STEP 2: Acupressure Point Li4 - This point is forbidden for pregnant women - *Start with a less painful side*

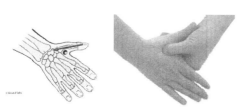

Location: between thumb and index finger as indicated on the picture.

Direction: apply firm deep strokes of pressure in upward direction. The initial painful sensation will soon begin to subside.

Duration: 2 min

STEP 3: Acupressure Point Li4 - This point is forbidden for pregnant women - *Switch to a more painful side*

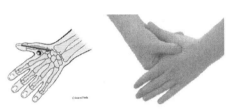

Location: between thumb and index finger as indicated on the picture.

Direction: apply firm deep strokes of pressure in upward direction. The initial painful sensation will soon begin to subside.

Duration: 2 min

STEP 4: Acupressure Point St36 - This point is forbidden for pregnant women - *Start with a less painful side*

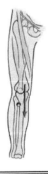

Location: with the tip of your index finger probe the area on the front side of a leg below the knee until you feel a slight dip.

Direction: apply firm deep strokes of pressure in downward direction. The initial painful sensation will soon begin to subside.

Duration: 1 min

STEP 5: Acupressure Point St36 - This point is forbidden for pregnant women - *Switch to a more painful side*

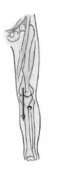

Location: with the tip of your index finger probe the area on the front side of a leg below the knee until you feel a slight dip.

Direction: apply firm deep strokes of pressure in downward direction. The initial painful sensation will soon begin to subside.

Duration: 1 min

STEP 6: Acupressure Point SP6 - This point is forbidden for pregnant women - *Start with a less painful side*

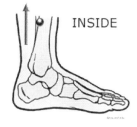

Location: on the inside surface of the leg, four fingers-width above the inner anklebone.

Direction: apply firm deep strokes of pressure in upward direction. The initial painful sensation will soon begin to subside

Duration: 1 min

STEP 7: Acupressure Point SP6 - This point is forbidden for pregnant women - *Switch to a more painful side*

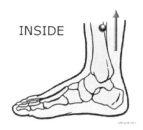

Location: on the inside surface of the leg, four fingers-width above the inner anklebone.

Direction: apply firm deep strokes of pressure in upward direction. The initial painful sensation will soon begin to subside

Duration: 1 min

STEP 8: Acupressure Point K1 - *Start with a less painful side*

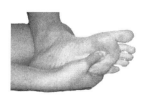

Location: in the center of the sole of the foot in the depression between the two pads.

Direction: if you are massaging this point yourself and cannot reach it, stand up with one foot on a tennis ball. Apply firm deep strokes of pressure in upward direction.

Duration: 1 min

STEP 9: Acupressure Point K1 - *Switch to a more painful side*

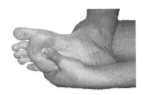

Location: in the center of the sole of the foot in the depression between the two pads.

Direction: if you are massaging this point yourself and cannot reach it, stand up with one foot on a tennis ball. Apply firm deep strokes of pressure in upward direction.

Duration: 1 min

STEP 10: Acupressure Point GB20 - *Start with a less painful side*

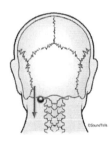

Location: just below the base of the scull, in the depression between the two major neck muscles.

Direction: apply firm deep strokes of pressure in downward direction.

Duration: 1 min

STEP 11: Acupressure Point GB20 - *Switch to a more painful side*

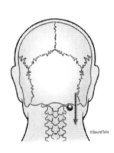

Location: just below the base of the scull, in the depression between the two major neck muscles.

Direction: apply firm deep strokes of pressure in downward direction.

Duration: 1 min

STEP 12: Acupressure Point Yin Tang

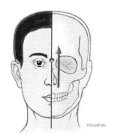

Location: with the tip of your thumb or index finger probe the area midway between the medial end of the two eyebrows as indicated on the picture until you feel a slight dip.

Direction: apply firm deep strokes of pressure in upward direction. The initial painful sensation will soon begin to subside

Duration: 1 min

STEP 13: Acupressure Point K27 - *Start with a less painful side*

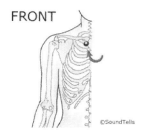

FRONT

Location: in the hollow under the clavicle, next to the breastbone. To find the point follow the clavicle until it connects to the breastbone. If you have difficulty following the clavicle bone, move shoulder back and forth.

Direction: apply firm deep strokes of pressure into the chest.

Duration: 1 min

STEP 14: Acupressure Point K27 - *Switch to a more painful side*

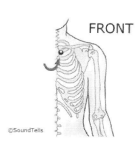

FRONT

Location: in the hollow under the clavicle, next to the breastbone. To find the point follow the clavicle until it connects to the breastbone. If you have difficulty following the clavicle bone, move shoulder back and forth.

Direction: apply firm deep strokes of pressure into the chest.

Duration: 1 min

123

Acupressure During Pregnancy

Morning sickness is likely due to hormones released by your body (estrogens). The symptoms include nausea and vomiting. These tend to be worst in the morning but can occur at any time of the day or night. Morning sickness is limited to the first trimester in the majority of women. Acupressure is often very effective method to relieve morning sickness.

Diet

Ginger is effective remedy for morning sickness. You can take ground ginger in capsules, use ginger as a tea, or take ginger chunks covered with sugar.

General advise for reducing morning sickness symptoms

- ❏ Get lots of sleep.
- ❏ An empty stomach usually worsens nausea. Eating several small meals will keep your stomach full and reduce nausea.
- ❏ To avoid vomiting in the morning eat something while in the bed.
- ❏ Avoid iron supplements, which may worsen nausea. Iron supplements are not necessary during the first trimester.
- ❏ Reduce fatty food intake.

To relieve morning sickness, motion sickness, and nausea, massage point P6 for as long as you can:

Acupressure Point P6 - *Start with a less painful side*

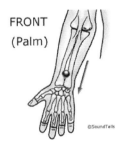

FRONT
(Palm)

©SoundTells

Location: on the interior side of the arm, in the hollow between the bones of the forearm, three finger-width above the wrist crease.

Direction: apply firm deep strokes of pressure in the direction of the palm. The initial painful sensation will soon begin to subside

Duration: 3 min or more on each hand

WOMEN ONLY: *Acupressure During Pregnancy*

To relieve insomnia, nervousness and anxiety massage these points:

STEP 1: Acupressure Point B10 - *Both left and right*

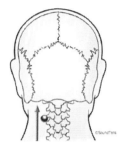

Location: halfway between the base of the skull and the base of the neck, on the edge of the trapezoid muscles.

Direction: apply firm deep strokes of pressure in upward direction. The initial painful sensation will soon begin to subside.

Duration: 1 min on each side

STEP 2: Acupressure Point Yin Tang

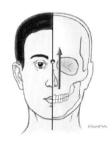

Location: with the tip of your thumb or index finger probe the area midway between the medial end of the two eyebrows as indicated on the picture until you feel a slight dip.

Direction: apply firm deep strokes of pressure in upward direction. The initial painful sensation will soon begin to subside

Duration: 2 min

STEP 3: Acupressure Point CV17

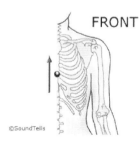

Location: in the center of the breastbone, midway between nipples.

Direction: apply firm deep strokes of pressure in upward direction. The initial painful sensation will soon begin to subside.

Duration: 3 min

WOMEN ONLY: *Acupressure During Pregnancy*

To relieve abdominal discomfort massage these points:

STEP 1: Points SP12 and SP13 - *Start with a less painful side*

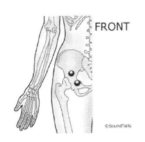

Location: SP13 (top) in the middle of the crease where leg joins the body (groin line), one finger-width up from the top of the pubic bone, four finger-width out of the midline.
SP12 (bottom) in the middle of the crease where leg joins the body (groin line), on the top of the pubic bone, three finger-width out of the midline.

Direction: apply firm deep pressure. The initial painful sensation will soon begin to subside.

Duration: 2 min each point.

STEP 2: Points SP12 and SP13 - *Switch to a more painful side*

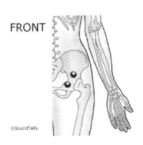

Location: SP13 (top) in the middle of the crease where leg joins the body (groin line), one finger-width up from the top of the pubic bone, four finger-width out of the midline.
SP12 (bottom) in the middle of the crease where leg joins the body (groin line), on the top of the pubic bone, three finger-width out of the midline.

Direction: apply firm deep pressure. The initial painful sensation will soon begin to subside.

Duration: 2 min each point.

WOMEN ONLY: *Acupressure During Pregnancy*

To relieve lower back pain massage these points:

STEP 1: Acupressure Points B27 to B34 - *Both left and right*

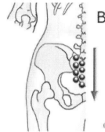

BACK **Location:** on the base of the spine.

Direction: if you are massaging these points yourself and cannot reach these points, lay back on a hard surface and position the tennis ball under the active points.

Duration: 2 min

STEP 2: Acupressure Point B48 - *Start with a less painful side*

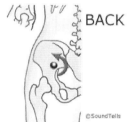

BACK **Location:** in the middle of each buttock.

Direction: apply firm deep strokes of pressure in upward direction. The initial painful sensation will soon begin to subside.

Duration: 1 min

STEP 3: Acupressure Point B48 - *Switch to a more painful side*

BACK 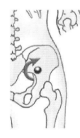 **Location:** in the middle of each buttock.

Direction: apply firm deep strokes of pressure in upward direction. The initial painful sensation will soon begin to subside.

Duration: 1 min

Urinary Problems:
Bed-wetting

Sit comfortably or lie down, close your eyes and breathe deeply when massaging the active points.

STEP 1: Acupressure Point CV4

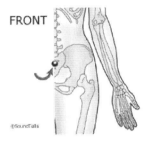

FRONT

Location: four fingers-width below the belly button.

Direction: apply firm deep strokes of pressure into the abdomen. The initial painful sensation will soon begin to subside.

Duration: 1 min

STEP 2: Acupressure Points K3 - This point is forbidden for pregnant women - *Start with a less painful side*

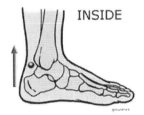

INSIDE

Location: in the hollow midway between inside anklebone and the Achilles tendon.

Direction: apply firm deep strokes of pressure in upward direction. The initial painful sensation will soon begin to subside.

Duration: 1 min

STEP 3: Acupressure Point K3 - This point is forbidden for pregnant women - *Switch to a more painful side*

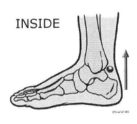

INSIDE

Location: in the hollow midway between inside anklebone and the Achilles tendon.

Direction: apply firm deep strokes of pressure in upward direction. The initial painful sensation will soon begin to subside.

Duration: 1 min

STEP 4: Acupressure Point SP6 - This point is forbidden for pregnant women - *Start with a less painful side*

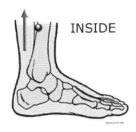

Location: on the inside surface of the leg, four fingers-width above the inner anklebone.

Direction: apply firm deep strokes of pressure in upward direction. The initial painful sensation will soon begin to subside

Duration: 1 min

STEP 5: Acupressure Point SP6 - This point is forbidden for pregnant women - *Switch to a more painful side*

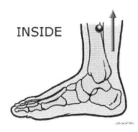

Location: on the inside surface of the leg, four fingers-width above the inner anklebone.

Direction: apply firm deep strokes of pressure in upward direction. The initial painful sensation will soon begin to subside

Duration: 1 min

STEP 6: Acupressure Point Yin Tang

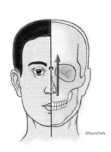

Location: with the tip of your thumb or index finger probe the area midway between the medial end of the two eyebrows as indicated on the picture until you feel a slight dip.

Direction: apply firm deep strokes of pressure in upward direction. The initial painful sensation will soon begin to subside

Duration: 1 min

Incontinence

Sit comfortably or lie down, close your eyes and breathe deeply when massaging the active points.

STEP 1: Acupressure Point CV2

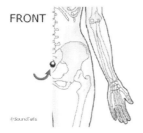

Location: palm-width below the belly button.

Direction: apply firm deep strokes of pressure into the abdomen. The initial painful sensation will soon begin to subside.

Duration: 1 min

STEP 2: Acupressure Point SP6 - This point is forbidden for pregnant women - *Start with a less painful side*

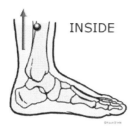

Location: on the inside surface of the leg, four fingers-width above the inner anklebone.

Direction: apply firm deep strokes of pressure in upward direction. The initial painful sensation will soon begin to subside

Duration: 1 min

STEP 3: Acupressure Point SP6 - This point is forbidden for pregnant women - *Switch to a more painful side*

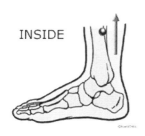

Location: on the inside surface of the leg, four fingers-width above the inner anklebone.

Direction: apply firm deep strokes of pressure in upward direction. The initial painful sensation will soon begin to subside

Duration: 1 min

STEP 4: Acupressure Point TW15 - *Start with a less painful side*

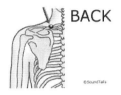

Location: on the top of the shoulder blade. To find the point go directly up from the nipple, around the top of the trapezoid muscle, and down to the top of the shoulder blade.

Direction: apply firm deep strokes of pressure in upward direction. The initial painful sensation will soon begin to subside

Duration: 1 min

STEP 5: Acupressure Point TW15 - *Switch to a more painful side*

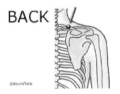

Location: on the top of the shoulder blade. To find the point go directly up from the nipple, around the top of the trapezoid muscle, and down to the top of the shoulder blade.

Direction: apply firm deep strokes of pressure in upward direction. The initial painful sensation will soon begin to subside

Duration: 1 min

STEP 6: Acupressure Point Yin Tang

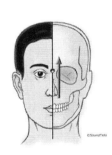

Location: with the tip of your thumb or index finger probe the area midway between the medial end of the two eyebrows as indicated on the picture until you feel a slight dip.

Direction: apply firm deep strokes of pressure in upward direction. The initial painful sensation will soon begin to subside

Duration: 1 min

Urinary Retention

Sit comfortably or lie down, close your eyes and breathe deeply when massaging the active points.

STEP 1: Acupressure Point SP9 - *both left and right*

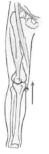

Location: on the inside of the leg, under the kneecap in the hollow just below the bulge.

Direction: apply firm deep strokes of pressure in upward direction. The initial painful sensation will soon begin to subside.

Duration: 1 min

STEP 2: Acupressure Point SP6 - This point is forbidden for pregnant women - *Start with a less painful side*

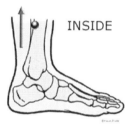

INSIDE

Location: on the inside surface of the leg, four fingers-width above the inner anklebone.

Direction: apply firm deep strokes of pressure in upward direction. The initial painful sensation will soon begin to subside

Duration: 1 min

STEP 3: Acupressure Point SP6 - This point is forbidden for pregnant women - *Switch to a more painful side*

INSIDE

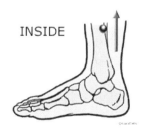

Location: on the inside surface of the leg, four fingers-width above the inner anklebone.

Direction: apply firm deep strokes of pressure in upward direction. The initial painful sensation will soon begin to subside

Duration: 1 min

STEP 4: Acupressure Point TW15 - *Start with a less painful side*

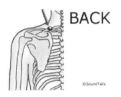

Location: on the top of the shoulder blade. To find the point go directly up from the nipple, around the top of the trapezoid muscle, and down to the top of the shoulder blade.

Direction: apply firm deep strokes of pressure in upward direction. The initial painful sensation will soon begin to subside

Duration: 1 min

STEP 5: Acupressure Point TW15 - *Switch to a more painful side*

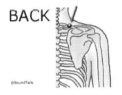

Location: on the top of the shoulder blade. To find the point go directly up from the nipple, around the top of the trapezoid muscle, and down to the top of the shoulder blade.

Direction: apply firm deep strokes of pressure in upward direction. The initial painful sensation will soon begin to subside

Duration: 1 min

STEP 6: Acupressure Point Yin Tang

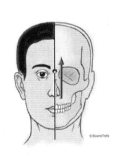

Location: with the tip of your thumb or index finger probe the area midway between the medial end of the two eyebrows as indicated on the picture until you feel a slight dip.

Direction: apply firm deep strokes of pressure in upward direction. The initial painful sensation will soon begin to subside

Duration: 1 min

Other:
Nose Bleeding

Sit comfortably or lie down, close your eyes and breathe deeply when massaging the active points.

STEP 1: Acupressure Point GV26

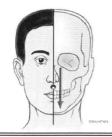

Location: in the hollow between the upper lip and the nose.

Direction: apply firm deep strokes of pressure in downward direction. The initial painful sensation will soon begin to subside.

Duration: 1 min

STEP 2: Acupressure Point GB20 - *Start with a less painful side*

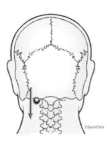

Location: just below the base of the scull, in the depression between the two major neck muscles.

Direction: apply firm deep strokes of pressure in downward direction.

Duration: 1 min

STEP 3: Acupressure Point GB20 - *Switch to a more painful side*

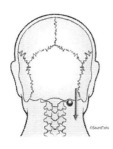

Location: just below the base of the scull, in the depression between the two major neck muscles.

Direction: apply firm deep strokes of pressure in downward direction.

Duration: 1 min

STEP 4: Acupressure Point P6 - *Start with a less painful side*

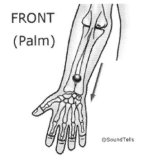

FRONT
(Palm)

Location: on the interior side of the arm, in the hollow between the bones of the forearm, three finger-width above the wrist crease.

Direction: apply firm deep strokes of pressure in the direction of the palm. The initial painful sensation will soon begin to subside

Duration: 3 min or more

STEP 5: Acupressure Point P6 - *Switch to a more painful side*

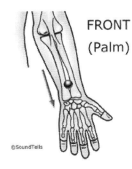

FRONT
(Palm)

Location: on the interior side of the arm, in the hollow between the bones of the forearm, three finger-width above the wrist crease.

Direction: apply firm deep strokes of pressure in the direction of the palm. The initial painful sensation will soon begin to subside

Duration: 3 min or more

STEP 6: Acupressure Point Li4 - This point is forbidden for pregnant women - *Start with a less painful side*

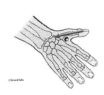
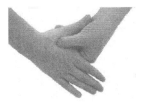

Location: between thumb and index finger as indicated on the picture.

Direction: apply firm deep strokes of pressure in upward direction.

Duration: 2 min on the left hand and 2 min on the right hand

Itching

Acupressure is often successful in reducing itching. Sit comfortably or lie down, close your eyes and breathe deeply when massaging the active points.

STEP 1: Acupressure Point Li11 - *Start with a less painful side*

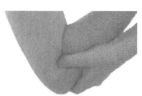

Location: bend your arm, press your thumb into the hollow located on the outer side of the arm, directly above the elbow, between the elbow joint (below) and the muscle (above).

Direction: apply firm deep strokes of pressure in the direction of the elbow joint. The initial painful sensation will soon begin to subside.

Duration: 1 min

STEP 2: Acupressure Point Li11 - *Switch to a more painful side*

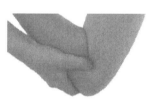

Location: bend your arm, press your thumb into the hollow located on the outer side of the arm, directly above the elbow, between the elbow joint (below) and the muscle (above).

Direction: apply firm deep strokes of pressure in the direction of the elbow joint. The initial painful sensation will soon begin to subside.

Duration: 1 min

STEP 3: Acupressure Point SP6 - This point is forbidden for pregnant women - *Start with a less painful side*

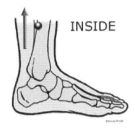

Location: on the inside surface of the leg, four fingers-width above the inner anklebone.

Direction: apply firm deep strokes of pressure in upward direction. The initial painful sensation will soon begin to subside

Duration: 1 min

STEP 4: Acupressure Point SP6 - This point is forbidden for pregnant women - *Switch to a more painful side*

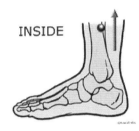

Location: on the inside surface of the leg, four fingers-width above the inner anklebone.

Direction: apply firm deep strokes of pressure in upward direction. The initial painful sensation will soon begin to subside

Duration: 1 min

STEP 5: Acupressure Point St36 - This point is forbidden for pregnant women - *Start with a less painful side*

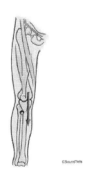

Location: with the tip of your index finger probe the area on the front side of a leg below the knee until you feel a slight dip.

Direction: apply firm deep strokes of pressure in downward direction. The initial painful sensation will soon begin to subside.

Duration: 1 min

STEP 6: Acupressure Point St36 - This point is forbidden for pregnant women - *Switch to a more painful side*

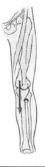

Location: with the tip of your index finger probe the area on the front side of a leg below the knee until you feel a slight dip.

Direction: apply firm deep strokes of pressure in downward direction. The initial painful sensation will soon begin to subside.

Duration: 1 min

STEP 7: Acupressure Point Li4 - This point is forbidden for pregnant women - *Start with a less painful side*

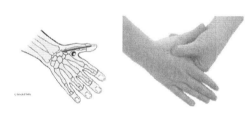

Location: between thumb and index finger as indicated on the picture.

Direction: apply firm deep strokes of pressure in upward direction. The initial painful sensation will soon begin to subside.

Duration: 2 min

STEP 8: Acupressure Point Li4 - This point is forbidden for pregnant women - *Switch to a more painful side*

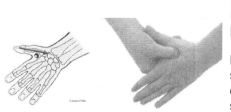

Location: between thumb and index finger as indicated on the picture.

Direction: apply firm deep strokes of pressure in upward direction. The initial painful sensation will soon begin to subside.

Duration: 2 min

Asthma

Asthma occurs when smooth muscles covering bronchial tubes contract increasing air flow resistance. Smooth muscles are controlled by hormones and autonomic nervous system. Acupressure is often a useful approach to asthma. Active points massage can be used during and between asthma episodes. Acupressure can be used in conjunction with bronchodilators.

STEP 1: Acupressure Point CV17

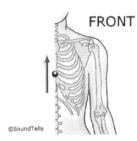

Location: in the center of the breastbone, midway between nipples.

Direction: apply firm deep strokes of pressure in upward direction. The initial painful sensation will soon begin to subside.

Duration: 2 min

STEP 2: Acupressure Point K27 - *Start with a less painful side*

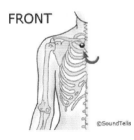

Location: in the hollow under the clavicle, next to the breastbone. To find the point follow the clavicle until it connects to the breastbone. If you have difficulty following the clavicle bone, move shoulder back and forth.

Direction: apply firm deep strokes of pressure into the chest.

Duration: 1 min

STEP 3: Acupressure Point K27 - *Switch to a more painful side*

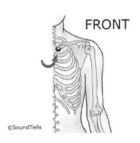

Location: in the hollow under the clavicle, next to the breastbone. To find the point follow the clavicle until it connects to the breastbone. If you have difficulty following the clavicle bone, move shoulder back and forth.

Direction: apply firm deep strokes of pressure into the chest.

Duration: 1 min

140

STEP 4: Acupressure Point Lu1 - *Start with a less painful side*

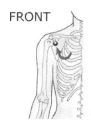

Location: on the outside edge of the rib cage, three finger-width below the clavicle.

Direction: apply firm deep strokes of pressure into the chest.

Duration: 1 min

STEP 5: Acupressure Point Lu1 - *Switch to a more painful side*

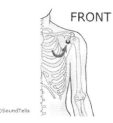

Location: on the outside edge of the rib cage, three finger-width below the clavicle.

Direction: apply firm deep strokes of pressure into the chest.

Duration: 1 min

STEP 6: Acupressure Point B13 - *Start with a less painful side*

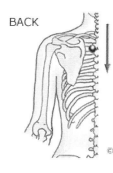

Location: between the spine and the shoulder blade, one finger-width below the top of shoulder blade.

Direction: apply firm deep strokes of pressure in downward direction. If you have difficulty reaching this point lay back on a hard surface and position a tennis ball under the active point.

Duration: 2 min

STEP 7: Acupressure Point B13 - *Switch to a more painful side*

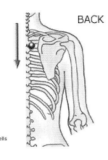

Location: between the spine and the shoulder blade, one finger-width below the top of shoulder blade.

Direction: apply firm deep strokes of pressure in downward direction. If you have difficulty reaching this point lay back on a hard surface and position a tennis ball under the active point.

Duration: 2 min

STEP 8: Acupressure Point St36 - This point is forbidden for pregnant women - *Start with a less painful side*

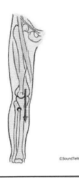

Location: with the tip of your index finger probe the area on the front side of a leg below the knee until you feel a slight dip.

Direction: apply firm deep strokes of pressure in downward direction. The initial painful sensation will soon begin to subside.

Duration: 1 min

STEP 9: Acupressure Point St36 - This point is forbidden for pregnant women - *Switch to a more painful side*

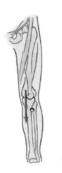

Location: with the tip of your index finger probe the area on the front side of a leg below the knee until you feel a slight dip.

Direction: apply firm deep strokes of pressure in downward direction. The initial painful sensation will soon begin to subside.

Duration: 1 min

Allergy

Allergies are due to overreaction of the immune system to environmental allergens such as pollen and dust. Acupressure treatment is often successful in reducing the symptoms. Treat as soon as first symptoms appear. Do not wait for full blown attack. Sit comfortably or lie down, close your eyes and breathe deeply when massaging the active points.

STEP 1: Acupressure Point St36 - This point is forbidden for pregnant women - *Start with a less painful side*

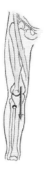

Location: with the tip of your index finger probe the area on the front side of a leg below the knee until you feel a slight dip.

Direction: apply firm deep strokes of pressure in downward direction. The initial painful sensation will soon begin to subside.

Duration: 1 min

STEP 2: Acupressure Point St36 - This point is forbidden for pregnant women - *Switch to a more painful side*

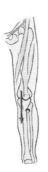

Location: with the tip of your index finger probe the area on the front side of a leg below the knee until you feel a slight dip.

Direction: apply firm deep strokes of pressure in downward direction. The initial painful sensation will soon begin to subside.

Duration: 1 min

STEP 3: Acupressure Point Liv3 - *Start with a less painful side*

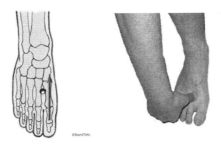

Location: on the top of the foot in the webbing between the big toe and the second toe.

Direction: apply firm deep strokes of pressure in upward direction. The initial painful sensation will soon begin to subside.

Duration: 1 min

STEP 4: Acupressure Point Liv3 - *Switch to a more painful side*

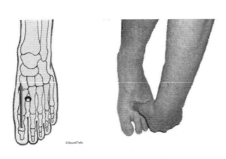

Location: on the top of the foot in the webbing between the big toe and the second toe.

Direction: apply firm deep strokes of pressure in upward direction. The initial painful sensation will soon begin to subside.

Duration: 1 min

STEP 5: Acupressure Point Li11 - *Start with a less painful side*

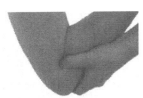

Location: bend your arm, press your thumb into the hollow located on the outer side of the arm, directly above the elbow, between the elbow joint (below) and the muscle (above).

Direction: apply firm deep strokes of pressure in the direction of the elbow joint. The initial painful sensation will soon begin to subside.

Duration: 1 min

OTHER: *Allergy*

STEP 6: Acupressure Point Li11 - *Switch to a more painful side*

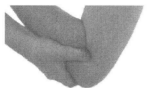

Location: bend your arm, press your thumb into the hollow located on the outer side of the arm, directly above the elbow, between the elbow joint (below) and the muscle (above).

Direction: apply firm deep strokes of pressure in the direction of the elbow joint. The initial painful sensation will soon begin to subside.

Duration: 1 min

STEP 7: Acupressure Point K27 - *Start with a less painful side*

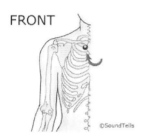

FRONT

Location: in the hollow under the clavicle, next to the breastbone. To find the point follow the clavicle until it connects to the breastbone. If you have difficulty following the clavicle bone, move shoulder back and forth.

Direction: apply firm deep strokes of pressure into the chest.

Duration: 1 min

STEP 8: Acupressure Point K27 - *Switch to a more painful side*

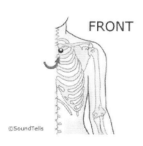

FRONT

Location: in the hollow under the clavicle, next to the breastbone. To find the point follow the clavicle until it connects to the breastbone. If you have difficulty following the clavicle bone, move shoulder back and forth.

Direction: apply firm deep strokes of pressure into the chest.

Duration: 1 min

STEP 9: Acupressure Point TW5 - *Start with a less painful side*

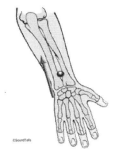

Location: on the back of the arm, in the depression between the two bones, three finger-width above the wrist crease.

Direction: apply firm deep strokes of pressure in upward direction. The initial painful sensation will soon begin to subside

Duration: 2 min

STEP 10: Acupressure Point TW5 - *Switch to a more painful side*

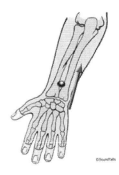

Location: on the back of the arm, in the depression between the two bones, three finger-width above the wrist crease.

Direction: apply firm deep strokes of pressure in upward direction. The initial painful sensation will soon begin to subside

Duration: 2 min

Decreased Libido Treatment

Decreased libido and impotency are commonly due to imbalance of autonomic nervous system. Acupressure can often be a useful approach to man's and woman's decreased libido treatment. Sit comfortably or lie down, close your eyes and breathe deeply when massaging the active points.

STEP 1: Acupressure Point CV6

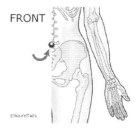

Location: two fingers-width below the belly button.

Direction: apply firm deep strokes of pressure into the abdomen. The initial painful sensation will soon begin to subside.

Duration: 1 min

STEP 2: Acupressure Point CV4

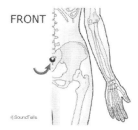

Location: four fingers-width below the belly button.

Direction: apply firm deep strokes of pressure into the abdomen. The initial painful sensation will soon begin to subside.

Duration: 1 min

STEP 3: Points SP12 and SP13 - *Start with a less painful side*

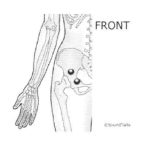

Location: SP13 (top) in the middle of the crease where leg joins the body (groin line), one finger-width up from the top of the pubic bone, four finger-width out of the midline.
SP12 (bottom) in the middle of the crease where leg joins the body (groin line), on the top of the pubic bone, three finger-width out of the midline.

Direction: apply firm deep pressure.

Duration: 2 min each point.

STEP 4: Points SP12 and SP13 - *Switch to a more painful side*

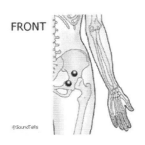

FRONT

Location: **SP13** (top) in the middle of the crease where leg joins the body (groin line), one finger-width up from the top of the pubic bone, four finger-width out of the midline.
SP12 (bottom) in the middle of the crease where leg joins the body (groin line), on the top of the pubic bone, three finger-width out of the midline.

Direction: apply firm deep pressure. The initial painful sensation will soon begin to subside.

Duration: 2 min each point.

STEP 5: Acupressure Point St36 - This point is forbidden for pregnant women - *Start with a less painful side*

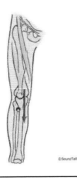

Location: with the tip of your index finger probe the area on the front side of a leg below the knee until you feel a slight dip.

Direction: apply firm deep strokes of pressure in downward direction. The initial painful sensation will soon begin to subside.

Duration: 1 min

STEP 6: Acupressure Point St36 - This point is forbidden for pregnant women - *Switch to a more painful side*

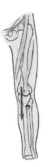

Location: with the tip of your index finger probe the area on the front side of a leg below the knee until you feel a slight dip.

Direction: apply firm deep strokes of pressure in downward direction. The initial painful sensation will soon begin to subside.

Duration: 1 min

STEP 7: Acupressure Point SP6 - This point is forbidden for pregnant women - *Start with a less painful side*

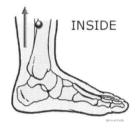

Location: on the inside surface of the leg, four fingers-width above the inner anklebone.

Direction: apply firm deep strokes of pressure in upward direction. The initial painful sensation will soon begin to subside

Duration: 1 min

STEP 8: Acupressure Point SP6 - This point is forbidden for pregnant women - *Switch to a more painful side*

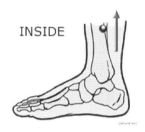

Location: on the inside surface of the leg, four fingers-width above the inner anklebone.

Direction: apply firm deep strokes of pressure in upward direction. The initial painful sensation will soon begin to subside

Duration: 1 min

STEP 9: Acupressure Point K1 - *Start with a less painful side*

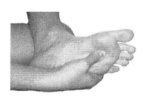

Location: in the center of the sole of the foot in the depression between the two pads.

Direction: if you are massaging this point yourself and cannot reach it, stand up with one foot on a tennis ball. Apply firm deep strokes of pressure in upward direction.

Duration: 1 min

OTHER: *Decreased Libido Treatment*

STEP 10: Acupressure Point K1 - *Switch to a more painful side*

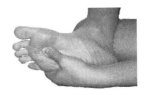

Location: in the center of the sole of the foot in the depression between the two pads.

Direction: if you are massaging this point yourself and cannot reach it, stand up with one foot on a tennis ball. Apply firm deep strokes of pressure in upward direction.

Duration: 1 min

STEP 11: Acupressure Points B27 to B34 - *Start with a less painful side*

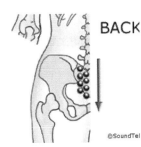

BACK **Location:** on the base of the spine.

Direction: if you are massaging these points yourself and cannot reach these points, lay back on a hard surface and position the tennis ball under the active points.

Duration: 2 min

STEP 12: Acupressure Points B27 to B34 - *Switch to a more painful side*

BACK 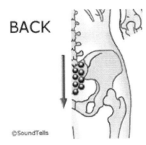 **Location:** on the base of the spine.

Direction: if you are massaging these points yourself and cannot reach these points, lay back on a hard surface and position the tennis ball under the active points.

Duration: 2 min

Hangover Treatment

Acupressure is an effective way to relieve painful sensation associated with hangover. Sit comfortably or lie down, close your eyes and breathe deeply when massaging the active points.

STEP 1: Acupressure Point Li4 - This point is forbidden for pregnant women - *Start with a less painful side*

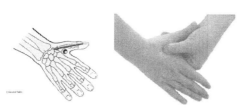

Location: between thumb and index finger as indicated on the picture.

Direction: apply firm deep strokes of pressure in upward direction.

Duration: 2 min

STEP 2: Acupressure Point Li4 - This point is forbidden for pregnant women - *Switch to a more painful side*

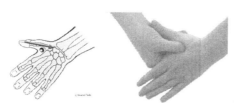

Location: between thumb and index finger as indicated on the picture.

Direction: apply firm deep strokes of pressure in upward direction.

Duration: 2 min

STEP 3: Acupressure Point GB20 - *Start with a less painful side*

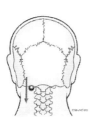

Location: just below the base of the scull, in the depression between the two major neck muscles.

Direction: apply firm deep strokes of pressure in downward direction.

Duration: 1 min

151

STEP 4: Acupressure Point GB20 - *Switch to a more painful side*

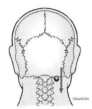

Location: just below the base of the scull, in the depression between the two major neck muscles.

Direction: apply firm deep strokes of pressure in downward direction.

Duration: 1 min

STEP 5: Acupressure Point GV20

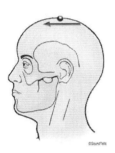

Location: with the tip of your index finger probe the area on the top of the head, where the line connecting the high points of your ears crosses the body midline until you feel a slight dip.

Direction: apply firm deep circular strokes of pressure in the forward direction. The initial painful sensation will soon begin to subside.

Duration: 2 min

STEP 6: Acupressure Point Tai Yang - *Start with a less painful side*

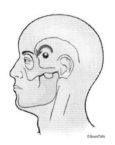

Location: in the large depression on the side of the head about 1 inch away from the end of the eyebrow.

Direction: massage in circular motions back to front. The initial painful sensation will soon begin to subside

Duration: 1 min

STEP 7: Acupressure Point Tai Yang - *Switch to a more painful side*

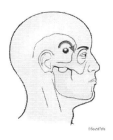

Location: in the large depression on the side of the head about 1 inch away from the end of the eyebrow.

Direction: massage in circular motions back to front. The initial painful sensation will soon begin to subside

Duration: 1 min

STEP 8: Acupressure Point St3 - *Start with a less painful side*

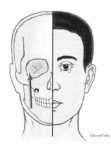

Location: below the cheekbone, directly down from the pupil of the eye.

Direction: apply firm deep strokes of pressure in upward direction against the bottom edge of the cheekbone. The initial painful sensation will soon begin to subside.

Duration: 1 min

STEP 9: Acupressure Point St3 - *Switch to a more painful side*

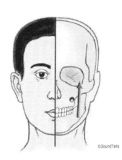

Location: below the cheekbone, directly down from the pupil of the eye.

Direction: apply firm deep strokes of pressure in upward direction against the bottom edge of the cheekbone. The initial painful sensation will soon begin to subside.

Duration: 1 min

STEP 10: Acupressure Point TW5 - *Start with a less painful side*

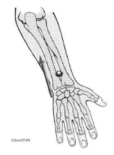

Location: on the back of the arm, in the depression between the two bones, three finger-width above the wrist crease.

Direction: apply firm deep strokes of pressure in upward direction. The initial painful sensation will soon begin to subside

Duration: 2 min

STEP 11: Acupressure Point TW5 - *Switch to a more painful side*

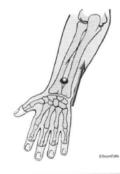

Location: on the back of the arm, in the depression between the two bones, three finger-width above the wrist crease.

Direction: apply firm deep strokes of pressure in upward direction. The initial painful sensation will soon begin to subside

Duration: 2 min

STEP 12: Acupressure Point St36 - **This point is forbidden for pregnant women** - *Start with a less painful side*

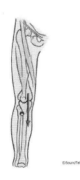

Location: with the tip of your index finger probe the area on the front side of a leg below the knee until you feel a slight dip.

Direction: apply firm deep strokes of pressure in downward direction. The initial painful sensation will soon begin to subside.

Duration: 1 min

STEP 13: Acupressure Point St36 - This point is forbidden for pregnant women - *Switch to a more painful side*

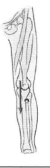

Location: with the tip of your index finger probe the area on the front side of a leg below the knee until you feel a slight dip.

Direction: apply firm deep strokes of pressure in downward direction. The initial painful sensation will soon begin to subside.

Duration: 1 min

STEP 14: Acupressure Point Liv3 - *Start with a less painful side*

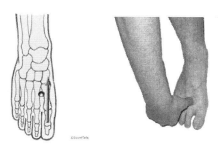

Location: on the top of the foot in the webbing between the big toe and the second toe.

Direction: apply firm deep strokes of pressure in upward direction. The initial painful sensation will soon begin to subside.

Duration: 1 min

STEP 15: Acupressure Point Liv3 - *Switch to a more painful side*

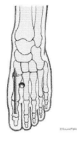 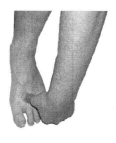

Location: on the top of the foot in the webbing between the big toe and the second toe.

Direction: apply firm deep strokes of pressure in upward direction. The initial painful sensation will soon begin to subside.

Duration: 1 min

Reviews

I am using the program to demonstrate the technique of acupressure to my patients.

I am a pediatrician, and often see patients with migraines, and I wanted to be able to offer something other than the usual Tylenol, Ibuprofen, etc. I am using the program to demonstrate the technique of acupressure to my patients.

A reviewer from Harrisburg

Excellent book! The major strength of the book are its crisp illustrations, thorough description of acupressure points location, and step-by-step explanations.

"Excellent book! The major strength of the book are its crisp illustrations, thorough description of acupressure points location, and step-by-step explanations. I have never tried acupressure before. I found this book very easy to use and very helpful in relieving my migraine."

Andrew Sharp from Austin, TX

Practical manual. Precise diagrams.

This is a very good manual, don't expect detailed explanations because there aren't. However, the diagrams are clear, precise and even though they are in black and white images they show everything that is necessary. I have no experience on acupressure and I can say that this manual is really useful. I have tried the explanations exposed here and to my surprise they really work! immediately, great, useful knowledge! Congratulations to the author.

Francisco from Mexico

I have read many different acupressure guides before. This one by far is the easiest to use.

I have read many different acupressure guides before. This one by far is the easiest to use. Finally, I can understand the location of points and duration of necessary massage. Thank you for this nice book.

Paul Stanley from Minneapolis, MI

Amazingly Simple!

Acupressure has been around for ages but as other holistic medical techniques it has not been a part of our Western medical practice. People usually resorted to it after everything else (drugs, surgery, etc) failed to help in their particular medical condition.
Clearly, simple, self-administered, drug-free acupressure techniques should be a starting point for treatment of any disease that is known to respond.
This book does not intend to give you a cure-all solution. To the contrary, the book (based on author's extensive research) gives you a "know-how" on addressing basic and common human medical problems that have been known since ancient China to respond to acupressure methods.

A reviewer from Boston, MA

I am no longer afraid of the headache!

I usually don't write reviews, but in this case I feel obliged to share my experience. I sometimes have this dull pain on the top of my head. Until recently I just had to survive until the bed time. Well, during one of those episodes I have downloaded the acupressure headache guide. Now I have used the guide on 3 separate occasions and I am no longer afraid of the headache. I had no previous experience with acupressure. So if this guide worked for me it can also help other people.

Marie Wilson from LA, CA

It sounds like magic, but the wrist pain ... disappeared after two treatments!

... I bought it to treat my carpal tunnel syndrome. It sounds like magic, but the wrist pain that bothered me for over 9 months disappeared after two treatments.

Barbara from Charlotte, SC

Excellent alternative approach!

I am not generally the type to resort to alternative medicine but found this book extremely helpful. Several months ago I began having migraine headaches and consulted several doctors who prescribed painkillers. That didn't help, plus I really didn't want to be taking such medication full time. Then I came across this book, which was recommended by a friend. At first I was skeptical but my wife insisted that I try the techniques and I eventually saw improvement. Although the headaches sometimes recur, I now know the techniques for managing them and don't feel the need for full time medication. Overall, I'd suggest this book to others who want to try to avoid doctor visits and tons of unnecessary medicine.

S. Lemberg from NYC

Good acupressure guide indeed!

Good acupressure guide indeed! ... Active point descriptions are easy to follow. I am using acupressure to treat my own and my son's migraines. I have also used acupressure to treat my neck pain.

Roger Green from London, UK

I am using this acupressure guide to treat my wife's headaches

"I am using this acupressure guide to treat my wife's headaches - she tells that it really helps her."

Paul Bauer from Cambridge, UK

Very well thought through collection of exercises!

Very well thought through collection of exercises! Very good artwork too. I was able to locate points with ease and my bad knee seems to be better.

Alex from LA, CA

Very comprehensive guide, good verbal description, great artwork!

I want to thank the developers of this software! Very comprehensive guide, good verbal description, great artwork, installs and runs seamlessly. I only wish this types of guides be available for other disorders.

Steve Shane from Washington, DC

I was able to alleviate my wrist pain!

My wrist was bothering me for over a year. I have tried wearing the splint but achieved little effect. My doctor was considering operation on my carpal tunnel nerve. I have decided to give a try to this Acupressure book. I was able to find trigger points indicated in the book easily - the description of the points was satisfactory. I have been massaging the points indicated in the book for several minutes each point. The pain subsided quickly after the massage. I have stopped treatment 2 weeks later. Now 3 weeks after I have stopped treatment I still have no problem with my hand.

Barbara from JP, MA

Made in the USA
San Bernardino, CA
21 March 2015